MANAGING SKIN DISEASES

PHILIP C. ANDERSON, MD

Professor and Director
Division of Dermatology
University of Missouri Health Sciences Center
Columbia Missouri

KRISTIN S. MALAKER, MD, M.S.P.H.

Clinical Instructor, Family and Community Medicine
University of Missouri Health Sciences Center
Columbia, Missouri

D1323498

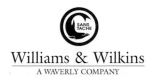

Williams & Wilkins
A WAVERLY COMPANY

BALTIMORE • PHILADELPHIA • LONDON • PARIS • BANGKOK
BUENOS AIRES • HONG KONG • MUNICH • SYDNEY • TOKYO • WROCLAW

Editor: Tim Hiscock
Managing Editor: Keith Murphy
Marketing Manager: Daniell Griffin

351 West Camden Street
Baltimore, Maryland 21201-2436 USA

The publisher is not responsible (as a matter of product liability, negligence or otherwise) for any injury resulting from any material contained herein. This publication contains information relating to general principles of medical care which should not be construed as specific instructions for individual patients. Manufacturers' product information and package inserts should be reviewed for current information, including contraindications, dosages and precautions.

Printed in Canada

First Edition, 1999

Library of Congress Cataloging-in-Publication Data

Anderson, Philip C.
  Managing skin diseases / Philip C. Anderson, Kristin S. Malaker.
  —1st ed.
       p.   cm.
  Includes index.
  ISBN 0-683-30598-0
  1. Skin—Diseases. 2. Primary care (Medicine)   I. Malaker,
Kristin S.   II. Title
  [DNLM: 1. Skin Diseases—diagnosis.   2. Skin Diseases—therapy.
3. Patient Care Management—economics.   4. Managed Care Programs.
5. Cooperative Behavior.   WR 140A548m 1998]
RL71.A48   1998
616.5—dc21
DNLM/DLC
for Library of Congress   98-25827
                                                                  CIP

The publishers have made every effort to trace the copyright holders for borrowed material. If they have inadvertently overlooked any, they will be pleased to make the necessary arrangements at the first opportunity.
  To purchase additional copies of this book, call our customer service department at **(800) 638-0672** or fax orders to **(800) 447-8438**. For other book services, including chapter reprints and large quantity sales, ask for the Special Sales department.

  Canadian customers should call **(800) 665-1148**, or fax **(800) 665-0103**. For all other calls originating outside of the United States, please call **(410) 528-4223** or fax us at **(410) 528-8550**.

  Visit Williams & Wilkins on the Internet: http://www.wwilkins.com or contact our customer service department at custserv@wwilkins.com. Williams & Wilkins customer service representatives are available from 8:30 am to 6:00 pm, EST, Monday through Friday, for telephone access.

99 00 01 02
1 2 3 4 5 6 7 8 9 10

ACKNOWLEDGMENTS

We are indebted to those hundreds of medical students and dozens of residents at our university who have tried out our ideas, in their training and in their practices over the last decade. In the last three years, faculty and residents in Family Practice and in Dermatology read and re-read drafts of the chapters of this book to be sure that what we practiced was what we preached. Practitioners and residents at Southern Illinois University, St. John's Hospital in St. Louis, and Tulane University also reviewed sections of the book.

Without the patient day-to-day labor of Mrs. Cinda Cannon, our scattered raw materials would never have come together as a book. To all these collaborators, we are grateful.

Contents

PART III
SPECIAL POPULATIONS

HOW TO USE THIS BOOK

This book is concerned with the management of patients who have diseases of the skin. It is concerned particularly with curing them or improving their disease quickly with the least possible waste of money and resources. Because only a finite amount of the nation's time/money/resources can be expended on medical care, efficiency is *required* if excellent medical care is to be provided eventually to a majority of our citizens. The pursuit of efficiency is a noble and professional goal for all physicians.

In our decade of experience with collaborative dermatology, the key to success has been to frame the problem from the primary care viewpoint, and then examine it together. We look at both quality of service and at all the costs, including money, delay, and awkwardness in the clinic. Primarily, the result should benefit the patient. No useless therapy. All of this collaborative planning is done prior to and apart from the usual case-by-case consultations. Patients should not have to play the specialist against the primary provider, if the two have a system of care on which they are agreed. Patients would recognize the collaboration as sufficiently good care. This book presents a model system that we have been working with for a decade.

To collaborate, the physicians must do an analysis of their clinical performance, including costs. Our system deals with the excessive costs of insufficient diagnosis, unnecessary biopsies, elective surgery, unproven therapy, and cosmetic treatments. The dermatologist must not be a "court of appeal" for the patient to obtain services not provided in the medical care agreement or not advised by the primary care provider. Collaboration prevents this argument and creates good patient relations. The family doctor ought to have an optimal situation in which to solve the problem on the first visit.

In collaboration, it is *necessary* to agree generally on the methods and language of diagnosis and treatment so that consultation usually can be done on the spot, simply, by telephone, fax, or telemedicine, without the burden of another visit to the dermatologist. On-the-spot consultation demonstrates to the patient that the two physicians are skilled, co-operating, and in full agreement. The number of old-fashioned double-visits, first to the family practitioner, then, with another appointment, to the dermatologist, needs to be reduced to a minimum. To make this reduction a set of shared decisions about how to care for skin disease must be accepted. This book explains such a set of decisions.

Reducing the demand for dermatologic care while maintaining quality of care is an obvious goal. This can be done by preventive care, excellent patient education, instruction to patients for self-care, more use of nurses and physician-assistants in giving care, and in providing special clinics or services.

Toward this end, it is useful to SIMPLIFY care. Use fewer different drugs; use more shared routines of treatment. There must be a re-straint on individual doctors offering special "tricks" or unique treatments to attract patients. Everyone must do the same basic essential treatments.

For instance, a tight audit is necessary on useless biopsies because biopsies are very expensive, use extensive resources, and require the time of the top decision makers. To surgically remove most of the harmless "lumps and bumps" in the skin of patients is *not* medically useful and is very costly. Collaborative restraint is needed, with prior agreement among the physicians and openness with the patients.

Obviously, physicians must give up some of their independence to do collaborative medicine. If their pride is wounded, they won't be effective. For example, all grade-four acne patients should be sent immediately to the dermatologist without any trials of antibiotics first. The dermatologist can coordinate the needed medical and surgical care more efficiently with fewer and shorter visits, which saves money for the doctor in capitated care and for the patient in costs of enrollment in the plan. Waste is good for no one.

Some collaborative groups may want to use a different style of dividing up the cases than we do. One approach is to have a local primary care expert. We encourage someone in each primary care group to cultivate a special interest in dermatology and to organize the clinic resources and staff to do more procedures quickly and efficiently. This person might be the liaison with the dermatologist, managing the performance audits, histopathology, and analysis of problem cases. The guidelines we present in our book are well tested during years of practice, but other arrangements would be feasible, provided they meet the two tests of quality and efficiency.

The prevention of major surgery at great expense for advanced skin cancer is another goal of collaborative care that focuses on finding and treating precancer of the skin. Similarly, the prevention of non-healing leg ulcers or diabetic necrosis in toes is a feasible goal in collaborative medicine. The failure to prevent progression of tractable medical conditions into expensive problems is a proper line of performance audit for the physicians. We need to prevent the waste in inadequate early medical care. Incentives for the patients to cooperate in preventive medicine can be built into the enrollment costs.

Our book is a primer in collaborative care, useful to nurses, physician assistants, telemedicine staffs, and many others. Physicians who have operated alone in private offices may find the adjustment to a more efficient cooperative system awkward. Experience shows us that most will appreciate the many benefits. Collaborative medicine has a promising future. This book, based on a decade of experience, is a good beginning.

PART I

Introduction to Primary Care Dermatology

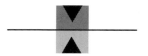

CHAPTER 1

MANAGED CARE

Today, physicians are concerned about practicing quality medicine within the tight financial limits of cost control imposed by managed care corporations. Traditional fee-for-service medical practice reigned until the late 1980s when capitation became increasingly prevalent. In the "good old days," the physician was not significantly concerned with cost of care. The money charged for patient visits and procedures was directly and proportionally related to the physician's income. A physician could provide any service, in any facility, as the patient care market demanded. Therapies and procedures were all paid for in the fee-for-service model. Such reimbursement occurred regardless of the overall necessity of the ordered treatment or diagnostic test in the management of the specific disease process. This health care system of the past included no incentive to reduce possible waste, error, or inefficiency.

In fee-for-service medical practice, physicians worked in mutual autonomy. Primary care practitioners performed general patient care and were not reluctant to refer to a specialist because there was no incentive not to do so. Also, patients could choose to present to a specialist with a problem without first having to get a formal referral from their primary care practitioner. This environment encouraged physicians to work alone, with communication based on referrals. Both offices would get paid, and there was no monetary incentive not to send the patient in question. No attempt was made to manage the patient's problem without referring the individual for a separate appointment with the specialist. Such collaboration in the fee-for-service model would only require more time spent by both physicians with less overall reimbursement for either party. Seldom did they develop collaborative methods of patient care. Collaboration would have been momentarily counterproductive.

The fee-for-service model of medical practice has quickly been replaced by capitated medical plans, most notably managed care. Managed care functions on the premise that, as long as quality patient care is being performed, less is more. The physician is encouraged to order only those tests and therapies necessary for appropriate diagnosis and treatment. A patient can see a specialist with minimal charge only if he or she possesses an official, formal referral from his or her primary care physician. Disease management should be performed with as few frills as possible. One such excess is unnecessary referral to a specialist. When they are functioning properly, managed care corporations reimburse the primary care practitioner based on his or her ability to provide quality patient care at the lowest possible cost. To keep charges at a minimum, referrals are discouraged unless wholly vital to the management of a patient's disease. However, regular evaluations of patient care outcomes must assure us that high-quality care actually is being delivered, and consultation is adequate to that need.

The system of managed care is extremely well suited for the development of collaborative patient management plans. This collaboration would exist between the primary care physician and the specialist. The two parties can study the fiscal feasibility of various therapies and the necessity of formal referrals. The costs and the benefits of each approach to commonly encountered medical ailments could be studied and agreed upon. The collaboration would need to occur in an on-going basis with constant scrutiny to ensure quality patient care is wholly maintained. In the best situation, both physician parties are aware of the rules of referral for each common disease process before the specific ailment presents itself at the level of the primary care clinic. Secrecy between physicians about real costs and medical decisions would be destructive to the overall reimbursement physicians obtain—not to mention its negative impact on providing quality medical care to the patient. Success in managed care requires strong collaboration, openness, and honesty between physicians. Physicians working autonomously in a managed care environment are performing a disservice to both the patient and themselves.

When competently managed, medical care ought to be attractive to both the consumer and the physician in regard to the premier issue of quality. When quality care is as important as cost containment, we can expect the demand for services to soar. In this environment, physicians can enjoy satisfying and productive careers. Collaboration between physicians in the management of disease supports the issue of quality of care without raising concerns about increasing the overall cost of disease management. Thus, it affords an opportunity to perform excellent medicine and not sacrifice control of overall costs.

Although managed care has transformed the primary care physician's professional job description the most, this new approach to financial reimbursement of services has significantly changed the way all physicians practice medicine. Incorporating a collaborative approach requires input from both primary care and specialist parties. Devising such a system takes effort and time. But, the financial and quality-care rewards that can be gained by incorporating collaborative patient care enables the benefits of such a system to far outweigh the costs of its formation.

To successfully collaborate, the notion of consultation must be changed. The consultation between specialists and primary care physicians must begin before the patient visits. The two physicians are partners in making a commitment to planning and incorporating the collaborative system. The idea of "autonomy" in physician practice fades into a new mutual effort at improving the quality of our current health care system. This book is a vigorous effort to promote these new ideas in the management of patients and their skin disease.

At the University of Missouri, the departments of family and community medicine and dermatology have spent many years working the kinks out of a system of collaboration. Our departments have successfully incorporated mutual collaboration in patient care. To this end, we have employed the aid of numerous residents-in-training and teaching faculty in both our departments. The efforts have been rewarding for both the family practitioners and the dermatologists. Our system of collaborative approach to patient care employs open communication via phone conferencing and/or telemedicine consults at the time the patient is being seen in the primary care clinic. Thus, the physicians involved can confer on the patient's clinical presentation, and all pertinent concerns can be personally discussed. If during the phone collaboration the skin changes are considered an emergency condition, the dermatologist will see the patient in the specialty clinic on the same day. If it is believed that the patient can be managed successfully without referral, tips on treatment and follow-up will be shared. It has been via this close departmental affiliation that we were able to devise the management focus of this textbook. The countless professional inquiries our physicians have dealt with together have enabled us to formulate a series of decision nodes for those skin diseases most commonly encountered in the primary care clinic. These decision nodes reflect when and how to treat these various diseases at the primary care level as well as when the patient is best sent to the specialist. Our history of ongoing collaboration and the wide acceptance we have received from both primary care practitioners and dermatologists has reassured us that both groups of physicians will find these management protocols helpful.

We first approached writing this book as a method by which to improve the training of the residents in both of our departments. We wanted the future practitioners to be aware of the importance of collaboration in the successful management of patients' skin disease in the modern health care market. We were also interested in the new approach to clinical studies generated by incorporating collaborative practice and working on simplicity in therapy. Although our initial intention in this book was to demonstrate the success of this systematic approach to clinical practice in residency training programs, we soon realized its potential in the private health care sector as well. Tests of its acceptability in non-teaching environments of both types of practice, dermatology and primary care, have proven that there is a wide market for incorporating the collaborative outlook that we have incorporated in this text.

CHAPTER 2

PROPER DIAGNOSIS OF SKIN DISEASE

As previously mentioned, to approach the diagnosis of a certain skin disease, the examiner must first determine the primary skin lesion that is present. But what are the possible primary lesions that may be involved? Primary lesions include the macule, papule, patch, plaque, nodule, vesicle, pustule, bulla, erosion, ulcer, and wheal. Now would be a good point at which to review the general language of dermatology. Our review of the language of dermatology in describing lesions follows:

> **Lesion:** any small area or disordered skin thought to be typical of the disease.
>
> **Rash:** also known as "the eruption," collection of individual lesions.
>
> **Macule:** small lesion with no substance on palpation (5 cm or less in diameter). Flat.
>
> **Patch:** big macule (i.e., greater than 0.5 cm in diameter).
>
> **Papule:** lesion that can be palpated and is 0.5 cm or smaller in diameter. It can be elevated, and it may be under the surface.
>
> **Plaque:** lesion that is palpable and flat-topped and greater than 1.0 cm in diameter. Plaques are papules clustered together.
>
> **Nodule:** round lesion that can be palpated and is greater than 0.5 cm in diameter; it is dome-shaped and not flat topped.
>
> **Vesicle:** blister, a fluid-filled papule (i.e., 0.5 cm or less in diameter). Fluid is clear or cloudy. If you break one, the fluid can be tested.

Pustule: fluid-filled papule, whose contents usually are white to yellow-white, the color of pus-exudate. Pigmented bacteria can modify the color.

Bulla: big vesicle. Bulla are greater than 0.5 cm in diameter and may arise from one vesicle that enlarges, the coalescence of many vesicles, or a large separation in the layers of the skin.

Erosion: shallow lesion formed by loss of just the overlying epithelium. Erosions arise from the breakdown of an overlying blister, or from traumatic disruption of the epithelium. Erosions don't scar.

Ulcer: lesion that arises from disruption of both overlying epithelium and dermis. It is deeper than an erosion. Ulcers don't form from the breakdown of blisters, but usually are due to vascular disruption or other direct destruction of dermis. Ulcers scar.

Nothing about skin disease is so useful in diagnosis and classification as is the primary lesion. All the possible primary lesions have been described above and should be employed when first approaching the diagnosis of an unknown skin disease. Remember, the symptoms of most dermatologic diseases vary and are too ill defined to base an initial differential diagnosis on them. Symptoms and patient history are helpful once the primary lesion has been determined. Again, the primary lesions are:

macule-patch-papule-nodule-plaque-vesicle-bulla-pustule-wheal-erosion-ulcer

Once the primary lesion has been determined the examiner can focus on narrowing down the differential diagnosis via looking for secondary changes. Such secondary changes include scale, crust, atrophy, and scar. The difference between scale and crust is that the latter are dissolvable in water whereas the former are not.

We can elaborate further on a rash by observing its color, texture, configuration, and distribution. Also, patient history should include some information about the sequence of the skin lesions. These important descriptors are outlined.

Color: Consider color only when you have recognized the basic structural morphology. Talk about color in simple terms of red, orange, yellow, green, blue, and violet. No one knows what ocher or magenta are. Further, define by saying "pale" or "dark" or "mottled" or "dense." Sometimes, color is crucial to diagnosis. "Pale violet lace-like" patches on the eyelids suggest dermatomyositis in children when there are no other skin lesions. Melanomas are shiny black. But, remember not to be so distracted by color that you overlook the primary lesion. Color is secondary in diagnosis, clearly less useful and less reliable than recognizing the primary lesion.

Texture: All lesions should be touched; and their overlying surface characteristics should be defined. This palpation is where crust, weeping, softness, roughness, etc . . . come into play. Palpation is especially important in diagnosing "lumps and bumps," as well as distinguishing between seborrheic keratoses and true skin cancers. Clinical training is most valuable in gaining experience with texture. Unfortunately, it is not a skill that can be picked up quickly or by reading alone. Talk in terms of rubber, rice grains, wooden, mushy, etc.

Configuration: The distinctive shape of individual lesions is the configuration. The language is about edges (margination), clusters, speckles, targets, rings, rosettes, lace-like patterns, homogeny, linear streaks, and other shapes.

Distribution: Skin diseases often have patterns over the body that are diagnostic and critical in defining the disease, for instance, the pattern of the fifth thoracic nerve segment in herpes zoster. With experience and clinical training, the patterns of various skin diseases become more easily recognizable. Learning these from textbooks is as elusive as is becoming aware of texture as noted. You can learn most easily in the clinic over time as you see new cases.

Sequence: Where possible, we would like to know when and how the lesion developed. Experience shows that patients are not skilled at reporting these changes and (most often) can be misleading. People often believe they have a "new mole" at a spot where photographs show a mole since age 12. Some claim they have "always had" a freshly growing basal cell carcinoma on their nose. It is best to rely first on morphology and use the history secondarily and cautiously, only to illuminate or support your morphologic diagnosis. For instance, in scabies, tiny itchy papules arise on the fingers or wrists that the patient may scratch off without being aware of the original lesions. Consider these further examples of typical sequences:

1. Allergic contact dermatitis: usually begins 48 hours after applying a contact allergen (i.e., neomycin cream) to the skin. Initially, the patient has the sudden onset of burning pain, and within a few hours, the characteristic vesicles and edema occur.

2. Irritant contact dermatitis: very gradual onset over weeks or months with much ebb and flow. As they become chronic, these skin lesions slowly, steadily worsen.
3. Seborrheic dermatitis: a lifetime of intermittent itching and scaling.
4. Psoriasis: long periods (months) of no change between short episodes (1-2 wk) of breaking out in the pattern distinctive to this disease. Lesions clear slowly, usually progressing from the center out towards the edges.
5. Herpes simplex: one or two days of distinctive stinging prodrome, followed by eruption of the vesicular lesions. Rash is often accompanied by malaise and lymphadenopathy. After 3-4 days of worsening, the lesions resolve within 5-6 days and may leave a thin scar.
6. Urticaria: arise quickly, but are migratory (not fixed) and resolve in a few hours, only to appear elsewhere on the skin.

Essential: Dermatologists may use the word "essential" together with a symptom (or sign) to signify that the symptom is present **without** any primary cutaneous lesion to account for it— "essential pruritus" or "essential melanosis" or "essential atrophy" are examples. Essential atrophy, for instance, would be atrophy in the skin not preceded by a disease that would account for the skin change.

CHOOSING ONE BEST WORKING DIAGNOSIS

We have discussed that the recognition of the **primary lesion** in skin disease is the key to correct diagnosis and proper treatment of a skin disease. Fifteen categories of disease, all based on the primary lesion, are listed. Although many other dermatologic diseases can be grouped in one of those categories, we mention here only those diseases that we determined were commonly encountered by the primary care physician.

1. Dry papulosquamous diseases
2. Eczematous diseases
3. Pustular diseases
4. Pigmented spots
5. Vascular changes
6. Lumps and bumps
7. Exanthem-like diseases

8. Acneiform diseases
9. Verrucoid diseases
10. Vesicular diseases
11. Bullous diseases
12. Focal necrosis of skin
13. Chancriform disorders
14. Heliosis
15. Urticarial diseases

These same fifteen groups are further expanded to include those diseases most commonly seen by the primary care practitioner which fall into each of these categories. Pick the best working diagnosis that fits the clinical picture of the skin disease in question.

1. Papulosquamous diseases
   a) Psoriasis
   b) Tineas
   c) Lupus erythematosus
   d) Pityriasis rosacea
   e) Lichen planus

2. Eczematous diseases
   a) Allergic contact dermatitis
   b) Irritant contact dermatitis
   c) Seborrheic dermatitis
   d) Atopic dermatitis
   e) Sunburn
   f) Scabies
   g) Dyshidrotic eczema
   h) Stasis dermatitis

3. Pustular diseases
   a) Pyodermas
   b) Pustular psoriasis
   c) Drug rash
   d) Molluscum contagiosum

4. Pigmented spots
   a) Nevi
   b) Melanoma
   c) Neurofibroma

    d) Lentigines
    e) Seborrheic keratosis
    f) Pigmentary changes

5. Vascular changes
    a) Erythema multiforme
    b) Ecchymosis
    c) Petechiae
    d) Vasculitis
    e) Vascular ulcers

6. Lumps and bumps
    a) Dermatofibroma
    b) Cherry angiomas
    c) Pilar cysts
    d) Lipoma
    e) Seborrheic keratosis

7. Exanthem-like diseases
    a) Measles
    b) Drug-rash
    c) Scarlet-fever
    d) Miliaria

8. Acneiform diseases
    a) Steroid acne
    b) Teen acne
    c) Rosacea
    d) Sarcoidosis

9. Verrucoid diseases
    a) Warts—verruca vulgaris, plantar, and paronychial
    b) Squamous cell carcinoma
    c) Actinic keratosis

10. Vesicular diseases
    a) Herpes simplex
    b) Varicella zoster
    c) Herpes zoster
    d) Fixed drug reaction

e) Scabies
f) Poison ivy–type allergic contact dermatitis

11. Focal necrosis
    a) Pyoderma—some herpes infections
    b) Venous stasis ulcer
    c) Venomous bug bite
    d) Diabetic ulcer

12. Chancriform diseases
    a) Syphilis
    b) Sporotrichosis
    c) Arthropod bite

13. Heliosis
    a) Poikiloderma
    b) Photo toxic rash
    c) Sunburn

14. Urticarial diseases
    a) Drug rash
    b) Hives
    c) Depositions
    d) Angioedema

15. Bullous diseases
    a) Pemphigoid
    b) Stevens-Johnson syndrome
    c) Bullous impetigo

CHAPTER 3

HOW TO EXAMINE SKIN, HAIR, NAILS, AND MUCOUS MEMBRANES

The key to success in clinical dermatology is the proper examination of the skin. To truly perform a thorough dermatologic examination, the skin must be closely observed and palpated. Once these skills have been mastered, the examination can be completely reliable when diagnosing skin diseases.

It is not necessary to mention the rudiments of physical examination of the skin taught in medical school, except to repeat that excellent lighting, magnifiers, and proper draping as well as the use of appropriate tables and capable assistants are important. Examining all of the skin is often necessary. It is a common diagnostic pitfall to look at only the one spot of skin that the patient shows you, when the patient is actually covered with other lesions. This mistake can cause a crucial error in arriving at the proper diagnosis. The patient may blame you for not doing the examination in the proper manner. Also, the physician should formulate diagrams, drawings, and even photographs of the patient's skin findings. These visual aids should be placed prominently in the patient's chart so they can be accessed as needed. Such documentation is crucial for follow-up visits and always helpful in the training setting.

Useful collaboration does require enhanced fundamental skills in the physical examination of the skin, hair, nails, and mucous membranes. Better examinations are needed because the collaborators must be confident that during phone and computer-based consultations, they are reliably discussing the same visible skin lesions in the same context. Mutual confidence rests on competence and precise recognition. This skill often includes the aforementioned diagrams, drawings, or photographs that should be used to facilitate quality review of a single patient's chart by several physicians.

Step back to gain an overall impression of the distribution of a specific skin change. This big picture is especially important in generalized rashes. The distribution and pattern of a specific rash is often typical of a certain skin disease. If possible, use your imagination to attempt to picture the pattern of the rash as a design. When attempting to determine the primary lesion again, be creative. Try to picture the primary lesion as if it were made of white wax floating in imaginary space. You will be surprised at how effective this mental imagery is in deciding on a primary lesion when seeing a mixture of skin changes.

Finally, consider "uncovering" some rashes by doing wet dressings, cleaning up crusts or fissures, and reducing infections. Removing a preponderance of secondary change allows you to more easily recognize the primary lesion that was previously obscured.

A brief outline of how to examine the hair, nails, and mucous membranes follows.

To Examine Hair

Examine the scalp for primary and secondary lesions just as you would hairless skin.

Look carefully at the scalp above the ears and in the nape of the neck, where infections and infestations often escape notice.

Look at the density of hair. Is the pattern regular?

Look at hair shape. Are the hairs thin, broken off, or discolored?

Plan to examine some hairs under the microscope, perhaps with your dermatologist.

Palpate the scalp for scarring, nodules, or infiltrates.

Note particularly whether eyebrows or eyelashes are involved in scalp diseases.

To Examine Nails

Look at all ten nails; not only the finger nails.

Nails grow about 3 mm a month, faster in youth, summer, on the dominant hand, on long fingers, and in hyperthyroidism. All kinds of febrile illness retard nail growth and may deform the nails.

The most common lesions of nails are onycholysis and subungual hyperkeratosis.

Onycholysis or white spots is splitting of the nail away from the nail plate. This separation is seen with any trauma or wet work. It can also be one cutaneous manifestation of psoriasis, eczema, and other common diseases of the skin.

Subungual hyperkeratosis is found usually with either psoriasis or onychomycosis. Do the KOH examination on the debris *under* the nail plate.

A variety of strange acquired and inherited disorders of nails do exist. Meet with your dermatologist to resolve these.

To Examine Mucous Membranes

Mucous membranes differ little from ordinary skin, except in the substitution of mucous glands for sweat glands, parakeratosis, and in the absence of follicles. Solitary sebaceous glands may be retained in the mouth and genital membranes as whitish-yellow papules, called Fordyce spots. Fibromas are common, due to trauma, and trivial vascular lesions can be seen and are normal. Palpate mucous membrane lesions to decide their thickness and texture.

CHAPTER 4

TREATMENTS

Designing effective, yet simple, systemic treatments for the most commonly encountered skin diseases in the primary care clinic was an essential part of our collaborative approach. As primary care physicians and dermatologists, we need to confer carefully and to agree on the therapy that should be employed for each of the skin diseases included in this text. We start with the primary care setting. We also sought to be able to explain these therapeutic approaches and the reasoning behind our suggesting them in detail to our staff and our patients. Treatments that are fads or fresh inventions without any evidence-based reasoning for their use must always be avoided. Our treatments follow logically from our presumptive diagnoses and were determined during our extensive collaboration. These agreed-upon therapies are a principal item in the quality of patient care.

In light of the above statements, each clinical group needs to put its own stamp on the therapy we have outlined in the chapters of this textbook. Each physician must review our recommendations and adapt them to his or her own collaborative group and his or her own level of dermatologic expertise. Then, they must choose the most feasible and financially sound approach. The option for referral to the dermatologist is always present in the event the rash cannot be classified or does not respond to the prescribed therapy.

For the purposes of this book, there are essentially only three groups of critical systemic medications to be used in treating the most common dermatologic diseases. These are anti-infectious agents (including antibiotics, antifungals, and antivirals), antihistamines, and corticosteroids. Of course, there are other valuable medications for various serious cutaneous diseases. Examples of such drugs include accutane, cyclosporine, dapsone, and methotrexate. These drugs are all used in serious forms of skin disease, are all associated with significant side effects, and are best used in prior collaboration with a dermatologist.

ANTI-INFECTIOUS AGENTS, ANTIFUNGALS, ANTIVIRALS, AND PESTICIDES

Antibiotics

Antibiotics are used to manage pyodermas. They function in the reduction of bacterial colonization of the affected skin. Those antibiotics employed for the majority of skin diseases act mainly via suppressing *Staphylococcus aureus* and *Streptococcus*. Other strains of bacteria rarely induce skin infection in the general population.

Thus, antibiotics of choice for skin infection with bacteria include those medications effective against *staph and strep*. Examples include:

>   Cloxacillin (500 mg) BID for 10 days
>   Cephalexin (500 mg) TID for 10 days

To treat *primary syphilis*:

>   Penicillin (2.4 million units IM) once *or*
>   Doxycycline (100 mg) BID for 14 days.
>   Remember the obligation to report STDs.

To treat *gonorrhea*:

>   Ciprofloxacin (500 mg) in a single oral dose

To treat *Rocky Mountain spotted fever*:

>   Tetracycline (500 mg) QID

To treat *acne*:

>   Tetracycline (500 mg) BID *or*
>   Amoxicillin (500 mg) BID *or*
>   Minocycline (100 mg) BID

To treat *rosacea*:

Tetracycline (500 mg) BID (with topical metronidazole BID)

Antifungals

Griseofulvin (ultramicrosize) is an effective and inexpensive option for many dermatophyte infections. Although it has significantly more side effects that its newer cousins below, griseofulvin remains the first-line treatment of choice for dermatophyte infections other than tinea versicolor and tinea unguium. Be certain to give the medication in the proper amount and do not underdose. Underdosing is the most common reason for failure of treatment. Griseofulvin should be taken with food to improve its absorption. The drug is not safe for use in pregnancy and is not compatible with anticoagulants.

Dosing of the antifungal is as follows. We use 330 mg of ultra-fine griseofulvin three times daily for full-sized adults. Give 7.25 mg/kg/day in three doses to children, always with food. Treatment must be for a total of 6 to 12 weeks in both adults and children. The main side effect with the use of griseofulvin is headache. One method to minimize headache is to either start the treatment with one-third dose and increase to full dose over 2 weeks or stop the drug for 2 days when the headache appears and then restart after this hiatus with a slowly increasing dose. Usually, either of these techniques is successful.

The newer antifungal drugs are expensive but are becoming popular due to their limited side effects. One such medication is terbinafine. This antifungal is the first-line treatment for tinea unguium and the second-line oral therapy for the rest of the dermatophytoses other than tinea versicolor. It has not yet been approved for use in children. Its effectiveness in the treatment of fungal nail infections is a result of its excellent ability to penetrate the affected nail. Unfortunately, the less expensive antifungal, griseofulvin, is poor at being absorbed into the nail and tinea unguium does not respond to griseofulvin. The dose of terbinafine is 250 mg each day in a single dose for 30 days total of therapy. Some studies have shown that it may require up to 90 days of treatment for some toenail dermatophyte infections. Terbinafine (250 mg BID) replaces griseofulvin for the treatment of inflammatory tinea in adults.

A third choice of systemic antifungal is itraconazole. The drug is currently recognized as second-line therapy for tinea unguium in the adult. But, it is significantly less effective against a fungal infection of the nail compared with terbinafine. Doses of itraconazole are 150 mg a day for 12 weeks total of therapy.

Antivirals

Antivirals are commonly used in the modern treatment of uncomplicated cases of herpes simplex and herpes zoster. They are also useful in treating cases of varicella zoster in the adult patient population. The medications are most effective in reducing the length and the severity of these viral diseases if given within the first 48 hours after the onset of symptoms or the outbreak of rash.

Recent trials with antiviral medications have shown valacyclovir and famciclovir to be as effective in oral doses as their older cousin acyclovir is in intravenous doses for the treatment of herpes zoster and varicella zoster infections. Thus, although intravenous acyclovir can be used to treat zoster infections, the advantage of the oral route of administration of valacyclovir and famciclovir is obvious. Interestingly though, oral acyclovir is nearly as effective in the treatment of certain herpes simplex infections and is lower in cost than oral valacyclovir and famciclovir. In treating the *initial* outbreak of *genital herpes simplex* infection, the medications of choice and the doses of these medications are as follows:

> Valacyclovir (1 g) three times daily for 10 days
> Famciclovir (500 mg) three times daily for 10 days

In treating *re-outbreaks* of **genital herpes simplex** infection or *any* **labial herpes simplex** infection, the medication choices and their doses are as follows:

> Valacyclovir (500 mg) three times daily for 10 days
> Famciclovir (250 mg) three times daily for 10 days
> Acyclovir (800 mg) five times daily for 10 days

Current practice in the systemic treatment of **herpes zoster** is more controversial. It is believed that the treatment is much more beneficial if initiated within the first 24 hours of symptom onset, but this advantage has never been proven via clinical study. The objective in the oral treatment of herpes zoster is to lessen pain and potential damage to the affected nerve root.

Valacyclovir (1 g) TID for 8 to 10 days
Famciclovir (500 mg) TID for 8 to 10 days
Acyclovir (5 mg/kg IV) daily for 10 days
(Oral acyclovir is significantly less effective than the above)

If an adult presents with the rash of **varicella zoster** within the first 48 hours of symptom onset, the addition of a systemic antiviral agent will often improve the course of this disease in the non-childhood patient population. Choices and doses are as follows:

Valacyclovir (1 g) TID for 7 days
Famciclovir (500 mg) TID for 10 days
Acyclovir (5 mg/kg IV) daily for 10 days
(Oral acyclovir is significantly less effective than the above)

Antihistamines

Antihistamines are an oral option for the treatment of urticaria and for the reduction of pruritus associated with various other skin diseases. Antihistamines are formulated into two distinct therapeutic classes—those that act on H1 receptors and those that act on H2 receptors. It is the H1 receptor antagonists that have the most therapeutic benefit in treating the pruritus associated with skin disease. Those antihistamines, such as cimetidine and ranitidine, that act at H2 receptors do NOT have important therapeutic actions on urticaria when used alone or on the pruritus associated with common skin diseases. Their principal use is as an adjunct to H1 antagonists in the management of chronic H1-resistant forms of urticaria.

It is the H1 class of antihistamines that are primarily employed in the dermatologic setting. Again, it is this class of drugs used in the treatment of urticaria and for the reduction of pruritus associated with various other skin diseases. Numerous H1 antagonists are available on the market. They basically are of two types—those with sedating side effects and those without sedating side effects. The *sedating* forms of H1 antagonists are the only type that effectively relieves pruritus in non-urticarial skin disorders. *Non-sedating* H1 antagonists can be helpful in urticarial skin disorders only. Examples of commonly used H1 antihistamines are listed below. The doses of these medications should be adjusted in a case-by-case basis.

Sedating antihistamines:
Hydroxyzine (25-50 mg) every 8 hours
Diphenhydramine (25-50 mg) every 8 hours
Chlorpheniramine (4 mg) every 6–8 hours
Cyproheptadine (4 mg) every 6–8 hours

Non-sedating antihistamines:
Terfenadine (60 mg) twice daily
Astemizole (10 mg) once daily
Loratadine (10 mg) once daily

Hydroxyzine has a known tranquilizing effect and is the antihistamine of choice in treating pruritic and urticarial skin disorders.

Corticosteroids

Systemic corticosteroids are overused in current dermatologic practice. These medications should be used only in those situations in which topical treatment has failed or the extensiveness of the skin changes makes topical therapy nearly impossible. All systemic steroids have side effects even when employed for short term usage. If taken for periods greater than 1 month, systemic corticosteroids can possibly lead to diabetes mellitus, hypertension, heart failure, hemorrhagic states, osteoporosis, infection, or the suppression of the pituitary-adrenal axis, thus supporting the judicious use of these potentially harmful medications.

Plan to become thoroughly familiar with just one oral corticosteroid and stick to using only that type when prescribing systemic corticosteroid therapy. Avoid the use of injectable forms, except in cases of emergent need such as anaphylaxis. The dermatologists systemic corticosteroid of choice is oral prednisone. The medication may be given in a burst or may be tapered over the course of a week to 10 days. The typical burst dose of oral prednisone is 40 to 60 mg once daily for 7 to 10 days. Then the medication is discontinued or re-evaluated.

There exist a few dermatologic conditions in which it is recommended we do *NOT* use systemic corticosteroids unless strong justification exists. These diseases include psoriasis, alopecia areata, inflammatory dermatophytosis, inflammatory herpes simplex infections, or pyodermas.

Some dermatologic diseases may require the use of high-dose systemic steroids for months or years. This administration should be performed in collaboration with a dermatologist. Obviously, such long-term use of high-dose systemic steroids will lead to the unwanted side effects associated with these medications. These skin diseases that may necessitate the use of high-dose systemic corticosteroids include chronic bullous diseases, systemic lupus erythematosus, dermatomyositis, severe vasculitis, severe acute conglobate acne, and a few erythrodermas.

In the long-term use of systemic corticosteroids, a thorough history and physical exam should be performed at the initial visit and at all follow-up office visits. When taking a history from these patients, the practitioner should pay special attention to the following histories:

1. Mental health disorders. Especially unusual anxiety, panic, depression, mania, eating disorders, alcohol abuse, and psychosis.
2. Peptic ulcers and related GI disease
3. Recent wounds, healing fractures
4. Bleeding disorders
5. Unstable diabetes
6. Heart disease—especially subacute bacterial endocarditis
7. Chronic respiratory disease
8. Recurrent or hidden infection
9. Adrenal or pituitary disease
10. Psoriasis

In the long-term use of steroids, a basic laboratory work-up should be done before the initiation of therapy. Laboratory investigation should include a CBC, SMAC, a chest x-ray, tuberculin test, TSH, and urinalysis.

Again, long-term systemic corticosteroid therapy is challenging and always risky to the patient's overall health. For this reason, the underlying diagnosis should be well established and peer reviewed before beginning high-dose or long-term corticosteroid therapy.

Topical Treatments

Many topical therapies will be presented in this text. Their function ranges from scabicides to simple lubricants. The individual drugs, their potency, the frequency of their administration, and the duration of necessary treatment will be discussed thoroughly in later chapters, along with the diseases which they are treating.

Finally, a quick review of patient education of *how to lubricate* is beneficial. Often, the treated skin disease does not remit, or is slow in doing so, due solely to lack of patient understanding of the method of lubrication.

When using any cream or lotion, the patient must apply one heaping tablespoon of the lubricant for each affected arm, leg, chest, and back (therefore, total body treatment would use 6 heaping tablespoons). Apply the lubricant to one extremity at a time and rub the material into the skin vigorously until all of the emollient is absorbed, and the superficial dead skin rolls off on your hands. Most skin diseases require twice-daily application of lubricant. More severe disorders need the emollient three times each day. The use of lubricants in children requires the same directions except substitute one heaping teaspoon for the one heaping tablespoon used in adults.

If using mineral oil, you can follow the same directions, but have the patient place old sweatsuits over the treated portion of their body for at least 1 hour after application. After this period, the patient may shower or bathe. Other considerations: eliminate high suds, like laundry detergents; we recommend Cheer free®, and use $^1/_2$ of the recommended amount of detergent. Also double rinse all clothing and bedding. Avoid all dryer sheets; if fabric softener is necessary, use one teaspoon in the laundry water per load. Remember to avoid long and/or hot showers as well as frequent soaping. Dove-free is a mild soap, and yet should be used sparingly.

Finally, a short note on the use of wet dressings. These dressings are both cooling and extremely antipruritic. They also help in the removal of edema and protect, clean, and splint the skin's surface. Wet dressings should be left in place for 15 to 60 minutes a treatment and may be changed once or twice during each application. Air dry the skin thoroughly after each wet dressing. This procedure will allow some of the associated edema to be removed. On an average, wet dressings should be used 3-4 times each day. The "wet" may be in the form of cool, refrigerated tap water or Burow's solution that is kept cool in the refrigerator to moisten the pieces of old bed sheets, torn into 1- to 2-inch segments. Patients may need demonstration of how to use the dressing. Burow's solution has a mild astringent effect that may benefit pruritus. Most patients who need wet dressings can followup with the primary care physician and need referral or phone consultation only if their conditions worsen or do not respond.

TABLE 1.1 ▼ Topical Corticosteroids

Superpotent	
Group 1	Temovate ointment or cream
	Diprolene ointment
Upper mid-range	
Group 2	Lidex ointment or cream
Group 3	Elocon ointment
Group 4–5	Triamcinolone 0.1% cream
Low-range	
Group 6–7	Triamcinolone 0.025% cream
	Hytone 1% cream

Use of Topical Corticosteroids

Simplify the use of topical steroids. Agree to use only a few.

Our approach is to use a mid-potency steroid cream routinely for all new eczema (Triamcinolone 0.1% cream) and a low-potency cream (Triamcinolone 0.025% cream) for long-term maintenance.

On occasion, super-potent topical steroids are used for the short term in a limited area under close supervision. We prefer either Temovate (0.05% of Diprolene), 0.05% ointment (Clobetasol, Betamethasone). Temovate is available in a cream and a solution for the scalp. For many situations, plain base can be substituted for low-potency steroid cream. Use this for "dry-skin."

If the variety of topical medications is kept small, efficiencies and cost savings result, time is conserved, and refills are easily done. Some adult patients with psoriasis like to use a high mid-potency ointment such as Lidex or Elocon, rather than Temovate for regular use. Strong topical steroids must be used carefully in children and older adults and not overused in body folds, on genitals, or on the face.

PART II

Disorders of the Skin

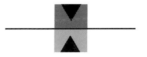

CHAPTER 5

MOST COMMON SKIN DISORDERS

▶ Acne Vulgaris

BACKGROUND

Acne vulgaris is a common skin disease. In fact, it affects more than 80% of all the people in the U.S. at one point during their lives. Roughly, 10 in 1000 cases of acne are severe enough to be disfiguring, whereas 300 in 1000 (if women) or 340 (if men) in 1000 have some acne that warrants prolonged medical treatment. Of these treatable forms, approximately 30% are mild cases and 10% are severe forms.

Acne is a disorder of the sebaceous hair follicle that occurs primarily due to a hormone-induced error in cornification, but with an additional variety of secondary factors that further the inflammation of the skin. The pathophysiology of acne includes three major mechanisms: the hereditary keratin defect with excessive sebum production, abnormal desquamation, and the presence of the bacterium Propionibacterium acnes.

Acne vulgaris has demonstrated a familial pattern of inheritance and tends to show similar forms in families. Thus, the patient's chart should include some awareness of those siblings and parents with histories of acne, preferably with the grade of each family member's acne.

Acne can be linked to hirsutism and various other hormonal disorders as well as to the use of medications such as isoniazid, anabolic steroids, bromides, depo-provera, norplant, and halogens. Thus, always keep these several etiologies in mind because these complicating etiologic factors also must be removed if acne is to respond to the treatment regimen that follows.

IN THE CLINIC

Acne lesions form within sebaceous follicles and can be papular, pustular, or nodular in form. More specifically, the variety of acne lesions range as follows: closed comedones (whiteheads), open comedones (black heads), inflamed papules, inflamed pustules, nodules, and cysts. Acne is best viewed and charted in regards to diagnosis and treatment if it is classified into one of the four "grades":

Grade I: Noninflammatory. Open and/or closed comedones.

Grade II: Inflammatory papules/pustules with or without comedonal lesions. No scarring.

Grade III: Deep and inflammatory. Edematous pustules and plaques. May also have above grade II lesions present. If severe ridges of lesions form with interspersed crypts and small nodules. There may be some early scarring. No large plaques no tunnels.

Grade IV: Deep and severely inflammatory with clusters of deep necrotic pustules forming furuncle-like lesions. Cysts, plaques, tunnels, ridges and nodules predominate. Always scarring. Grade IV may have scalp and axillary lesions and may be severe enough to become necrotizing in nature. Patients may become systemically ill.

DIAGNOSIS AND TREATMENT

Our treatment of acne vulgaris depends on agreeing on the aforementioned "grade." For example, using antibiotics in the treatment of grade I acne, as if it were grade III or IV, has no advantage. Never treat "above grade." To chart improvement in the patient, note changes in the grade. Explain to the patient that acne cannot be cured but can be controlled so the patient has reasonable expectations.

Grade I acne is entirely on the skin's surface and topical preparations manage the disease well. Topical treatment for grade I acne includes the following:

1. Retin-A at strengths of .025% to .1% applied to entire area of involvement. It is best to start at the lowest strength and progressively increase at 4-week intervals to minimize the drying and irritating side effects. For most patients, start with .025% cream at bedtime, applied approximately 15 minutes after

cleansing. Higher concentrations can be used once irritation is shown not to be a problem. Patients with extremely oily skin may prefer a gel form, which is more drying. Treatment requires 4–8 months for resolution of existing comedones. Maintenance is required to prevent recurrence, but need not be performed on a daily basis. Use the Patient Handout Information to teach the correct use of Retin-A. Because of popular concerns with the possibility of teratogenic affects, we avoid even these topical retinoids if the patient is pregnant.

2. Benzoyl peroxide preparations of 2.5%, 5%, and 10% are available as lotions, gels, or creams and can be applied once to twice daily, based on effectiveness. Mild redness is expected the first week of therapy. Benzoyl peroxide unplugs follicles and decreases number of P. acnes organisms. A 50–75% reduction in inflammatory lesions occurs within 8–12 weeks. Inform the patient that peroxides may depigment the skin somewhat in whites and more severely in darker skinned patients.

3. Other topical preparations are available over the counter. Unfortunately, many of these preparations have not been proven highly effective.

Grade II acne is still a surface form of acne, but the inflammatory nature often requires the addition of topical antibiotics to the above topical regimen of Retin-A and Benzoyl Peroxide. Topical antibiotics include erythromycin and clindamycin. These preparations decrease the P. acnes bacteria on the skin's surface, thereby reducing the unsightly inflammation. These topical antibiotics should be applied once to two times each day after cleansing.

Grade III acne is deep and can be mild or severe in form. Moderate grade III acne contains no scar, cyst, or tracts. Severe grade III acne is scarring, and small tracts, cysts, and ridges can occur, although they are few in number and moderate to mild in appearance. All grade III acne calls for long-term systemic antibiotics. The first choice is tetracycline 500 mg orally BID to QID. The second choice is Amoxicillin 250 mg orally TID. Other choices include erythromycin and minocycline; but these drugs have more side effects and/or are more expensive. Therapy must be maintained for 4–6 weeks before results are seen. Once this point is reached, you may taper the dose to once daily for maintenance. Recall that tetracycline is poorly tolerated if given at doses greater than 2 grams per day and should NEVER be used in pregnancy. Tetracycline and minocycline increase photosensitivity and thus the patient should be warned about exposure to sunlight while taking these medications. The addition of topicals, Retin-A and benzoyl peroxide, provide for relief of the superficial lesions that may be intermixed with the deeper lesions of grade III acne. If grade III acne is more severe, as described above, surgical treatment and injection is often necessary. These topics are discussed further below.

Grade IV acne (scarring, nodulocystic acne) requires personalized and aggressive therapy. This treatment includes oral Isotretinoin (Accutane), intralesional corticosteroid injection, and surgical incision and drainage of cysts or surgical excision of cysts and tracts. Accutane may be given at a dose of 1.0 mg/kg/day for 5 months of therapy. But, Accutane is a potentially dangerous drug that requires a large amount of time and experience to manage optimally. Not only is Accutane teratogenic, but it can cause arthralgias, hyperlipidemias, lipidemias, liver disease, and many other side effects. Surgery requires practice and is time consuming to the physician. Patients with severe acne will be quite anxious and concerned over possible disfigurement. Always remember to educate the patient thoroughly.

There are additional forms of acne that do not fall within the grading system of acne vulgaris. These variants include adult acne, steroid acne, contact acne, rosacea, and neonatal acne. These forms are discussed in the section "Rosacea, Other Acne" and thus won't be repeated here.

MANAGEMENT

To Manage

▼ Keep: All grade I and II
▼ Grade I—topicals only
   Retin-A—0.25% to 0.1% qhs
   Benzoyl Peroxide—2% to 10% qd to BID
▼ Grade II—above topicals plus:
   Topical antibiotics—erythromycin or clindamycin qd to BID
▼ Grade III without need for surgery
▼ Above topicals, Retin-A and Benzoyl Peroxide, plus:
▼ Oral antibiotics
   1st choice—Tetracycline 500 mg BID

2nd choice—Amoxicillin 250 mg TID or 500 mg BID

If no response: Minocycline 100 mg BID

If allergic: Erythromycin 500 mg BID

Decrease to qd after 4–6 weeks and clinical improvement

With all patients, emphasize control rather than quick cure—4–6 weeks of treatment before results are seen.

Send

▼ Grade III forms that are severe or quickly scarring (require surgery/injection)

▼ All grade IV

▼ Patients who do not respond to treatment in 8 weeks or any patient who worsens during therapeutic course.

Note: Surgery, injection, and Accutane administration are all time consuming, use special procedure set-ups, and usually require additional training, thus may be best handled in the managed care setting by a dermatologist.

PROGNOSIS

The prognosis for all acne vulgaris, if properly diagnosed and treated, is good. Vigorous therapy for 1–2 years is necessary in a few cases to maintain good results.

PEARLS AND PITFALLS

▼ Patients may cleanse with any oily skin formula facial soap (ex. Basis/Neutrogena) up to twice each day.

▼ Thoroughly rinse all soaps—unrinsed product may worsen acne.

▼ If acne distribution is not symmetrical, rule out chloracne or other irritant acne.

▼ Stress and diet are never factors in the development of acne lesions.

▼ Hot/humid weather and swimming in chlorinated water will worsen acne.

▼ Picking/squeezing should be thoroughly discouraged, will worsen all forms of acne.

▼ Modern combined BCP's do not cause acne (low progesterone levels), but progesterone only pills, depo Provera, and Norplant can trigger or worsen acne.

▼ When using cosmetics, employ oil-free and/or water soluble products.

▼ Watch out for pregnancy while treating acne with systemic antibiotics.

CASE STUDY

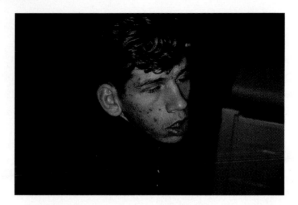

S: A 150-pound 18-year-old white male presents to your office with a 3–4 year history of "acne." He states the lesions are mostly superficial and not painful but occasionally he will develop a deep painful lesion on his chin, cheek or back. He is worse recently.

O: The lesions are present on his face, chest, and back. They consist of multiple open and closed comedones, especially near the nose, with many pustules and erythematous papules. Two deep nodules of $\frac{1}{4}$ cm in diameter do present, one in the left scapular region, the other on the chin. No scar is found.

A: Grade III acne—Superficial inflammatory acne with several deep lesions but no scar, fissure, tunnels or tracts and without evidence of scar.

P: 1. Oral antibiotic: Tetracycline (500 mg) orally BID or TID.
 2. Topical Retin-A to face q HS—start with 0.25% strength.
 3. Benzac AC 10% wash to back and chest once a day. Apply with long handled, soft brush and work gently into a mild lather.
 4. Recheck in 4 weeks.
 5. Explain—4–6 weeks to begin to see results. (Avoid long exposure to sunlight with use of tetracycline and Retin-A use).
 6. Patient need only to be sent on if the deep nodules do not show any response with oral antibiotics. Some lesions may require I&D, which is best and most cost effective if performed by a dermatologist.

PATIENT EDUCATION HANDOUT
ACNE VULGARIS

All acne products need 4–6 weeks to begin to display effectiveness.

The goal is to control and improve the skin's appearance. But remember, acne cannot be "cured." Hard work pays off in treating acne. Thus, follow your doctor's instructions.

Retin A use:
1. Causes severe dryness and flaking of the skin first 1–2 weeks of use. This side effect improves with time. It is often helpful to use a good moisturizer, such as Lubriderm or Cetaphil, the morning after Retin A application.
2. Apply Retin A at bedtime approximately 15 minutes after cleansing. If you apply it sooner than 15 minutes, absorptions is increased and the drying side effects are more prominent.
3. Do not use a moisturizer at the time of Retin A application. Again, this will increase absorption of the medicine and cause more dryness and flaking.

Topical antibiotics—apply a thin layer to only the effected areas one time each day.

Benzoyl Peroxide products—use as directed by the physician. If significant dryness and redness occurs, stop using and call your physician, you might require a lower strength preparation.

▶ DERMATOPHYTOSIS

BACKGOUND

For clinical purposes we have grouped all dermatophytosis and candidosis together because not only are they caused by plant-like organisms big enough to be seen easily with an ordinary microscope in a scraping from the stratum corneum, but treatment and clinical findings are similar as well. Dermatophyte infections are commonly known as ringworm. The infection can vary in clinical intensity, with lesions ranging in appearance from trivially scaly spots to highly inflammatory and pyoderma-like. These infections are best described in regards to their distribution: Tinea manum (hands), tines pedis (feet), tinea corporis (non hair bearing body), unguium (nails), and tinea barbae (beard).

It is not necessary to know the exact dermatophyte responsible for a specific fungal infection. Thus, the etiologic agent of each of the above infections will be discussed only briefly here. Tinea pedis, cruris, and manum are usually due to Trichophyton rubrum. Tinea capitis is caused by T. tonsurans in almost all cases. The possibility of skin infection developing secondary to these organisms is increased if eczema is commonly present or scratches are found on the skin surface. In other words, fungus invades damaged skin more readily than its intact counterpart. Also, since dermatophytoses flourish in hot moist climates, the disease is best cured in the dry, winter months. Summer months often require longer treatment courses.

IN THE CLINIC

The cutaneous morphology of the disease varies with the exact location of the infection. A few of the most common are as follows:

Tinea pedis usually starts with a fissure in the web space between the 4th and 5th toes.

Tinea manum is a non inflammatory scaling on the palm of the hand resembling eczema and usually occurs unilaterally.

Tinea cruris shows sharply marginated, red plaques on the upper, inner thighs and genital areas but never on the scrotum.

Tinea corporis demonstrates ring-shaped, erythematous lesions with varying degrees of central clearing and raised, scaling borders (often with tiny vesicles).

Tinea capitus is responsible for well-demarcated areas of hair loss, with the remaining hairs in the lesion demonstrating various lengths. Some underlying scale and inflammation of the scalp are always discernable as well. This form of dermatophytosis is seen mostly in children.

Tinea versicolor presents a small (<1 cm) macular spots of hypopigmentation or hyperpigmentation which enlarge and coalesce. Scale is always demonstrated on scraping with a #15 scalpel.

Pruritus is often an associated clinical finding in the patient with a dermatophyte infection. The amount of pruritus varies with the type and location of the infection. For example, Tinea pedis is extremely itchy, while Tinea versicolor is rarely pruritic. Tinea cruris (despite the common term "jock itch") is tender, not pruritic.

The differential diagnosis of dermatophytosis is extensive and varies with location of the lesion. Dermatophytoses may be vesicular and very inflammatory—often to the point of resembling allergic contact dermatitis or acute pyoderma. Severe symptoms of pain, malaise, and fever may occur with fungal infections, but are mostly demonstrated in the vesiculobullous or pyoderma like lesions. Tinea capitis can resemble psoriasis, seborrheic dermatitis, or lupus erythematosus. Tinea on the face can particularly resemble discoid lupus. Thus, it is always important to determine that the patient is suffering from a dermatophyte infection and not an eczema, psoriaiaform, or other dermatitis.

The easiest method by which to determine that the patient has a dermatophyte infection is via a KOH-examination. KOH examination is 80–90% sensitive and specific. It is most cost effective and efficient if this quick in-office test is performed and documented with the initial presentation of all suspected fungal infections. The proper method of KOH-examination follows at the end of this section. Often texts will refer to the use of Wood's light and its florescence to aid in the diagnosis of fungal infections. Unfortunately, most of the current inciting dermatophytes do not fluoresce under the wood's light; and its use as a diagnostic aid in fungal infections is outdated.

Most fungal infections remain superficial in nature, but deeper tissue layers can be involved. When seen at these deeper layers, the possibility of a concomitant bacterial pyoderma is increased. This finding is especially true of Tinea pedis.

Dermatophytoses of the feet are reliably linked to recurring cellulitis and other prodermas. Diabetic patients are particularly plagued with the secondary bacterial infections of Tinea pedis. Therefore, all diabetic patients with cellulitis or other forms of pyoderma of the feet and legs must be studied for dermatophytosis as a possible underlying etiology. This examination is essential if appropriate therapy is to be instituted quickly and effectively. Also, chronic leakage of bacteria through dermatophytosis of the feet is well proven and indicates the need to resolve any secondary substantial bacterial infection as well as the underlying fungal infection. Treatment of bacterial involvement may be especially necessary if erosion of fissuring is involved. Again, diabetic patients are a special concern and need to be vigorously treated and closely monitored.

DIAGNOSIS AND TREATMENT

The treatment of dermatophyte infections should begin after the following:

1. Confirmation of clinical suspicion via KOH examination
2. Clinically suspected fungal infection (other than T. capitus) with a negative KOH
3. If suspect T. capitus, and negative KOH, start treatment as below *only if* confirmation of dermatophyte infection via fungal culture (most cost effective if fungal culture performed by dermatologist)

Note: The reasoning behind the exception of not empirically treating tinea capitus is because the responsible dermatophyte does not respond to topical antifungal treatment and must be treated with oral antifungals, principally griseofulvin. This medication has potential serious side effects; these side effects in combination with the fact that Tinea capitus occurs mostly in children lends to the importance of diagnostic confirmation before initiation of treatment.

To treat Tinea corporis, manum, rubrum, cruris, barbae, and pedis, start with topical antifungals. Apply two times each day. Allow for a dry environment and eliminate all elements that increase moisture and occlusion. For example, frequently change socks, avoid vinyl shoes/boots, wear cotton liners in rubber gloves, use boxers instead of briefs, etc.

If after 2 weeks of topical antifungals BID the patient's skin changes do not improve, re-perform the KOH exam. If positive now, continue topical antifungal 2 times a day for 2 more weeks. If after 2 weeks, there is no improvement, initiate oral griseofulvin (330 mg ultramicrosize) in three divided doses daily. Treat for 2 weeks after skin changes resolve.

If the KOH exam after 2 weeks continues to be negative, it is most cost effective to send the patient to the dermatologist for fungal culture and consult.

With a patient who probably has Tinea capitus and a positive KOH, initiate oral griseofulvin therapy. Adult and child doses and treatment duration follows below. If the KOH is negative, proceed with a dermatology referral for fungal culture as previously mentioned.

If diagnosed with tines versicolor, the treatment consists of 5% Selenium Sulfide; apply at bedtime; leave on overnight; rinse thoroughly in the morning. The pigment changes can last up to 2 months even though the dermatophyte is no longer present. Any pruritus or scale will fully resolve with Selenium Sulfide treatment.

CASE STUDY

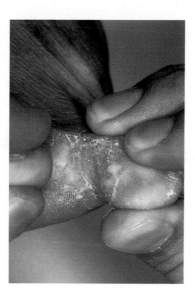

S: A 20-year-old mixed-race male basketball player for the Jackson Michigan Vikings presents with c/o peeling, itchy feet for 2–3 months. He admits to practicing for many hours a day in wet, sweat-filled socks. Many of his teammates are experiencing similar symptoms.

O: White macerated feet bilaterally with most marked changes in the web space between the 4th and 5th toes. Erosions are present. Marked excoriation is present. No associated erythema or edema. KOH performed—multiple hyphae with a few spores.

A: Tinea pedis (no secondary cellulitis)

P: Topical antifungal applied twice a day for 2 weeks. Recheck after 2 weeks. If improving, continue topicals until 2 weeks after full resolution. If no improvement, start oral griseofulvin in doses previously mentioned. Frequent sock changes—every hour if possible.

PATIENT EDUCATION HANDOUT
DERMATOPHYTE INFECTION

▼ Use the cream prescribed twice each day—morning and night.

▼ If your feet are affected, apply the cream to the entire bottom of the foot and the web space between each toe. Do this even if these areas do not show any skin changes. Remember to rub the cream in well to all areas, especially the creases.

▼ Foot powders are not recommended. These preparations can often irritate the fungus infection and make your feet feel worse.

▼ If any clothing touching the affected skin is wet/sweaty, change it. Wet environments will impair the healing of your skin infection.

▼ If prescribed a pill, take exactly as directed. Be sure to make all your follow-up visits/lab draws. These medications can have some serious side effects.

▼ If itching is severe, tell your doctor. He can prescribe a medicine to take by mouth for this problem.

▼ Be sure to avoid getting pregnant if you are taking a pill for your fungal infection—these can be harmful to your baby.

▶ ECZEMA

Eczema is the second most common skin disorder seen in the primary care clinic. The term "eczema" refers to a spectrum of skin disorders all of which are characterized by a micro vesicular skin reaction. The etiology of this reaction defines which specific type of eczema is present. Etiologies include allergens, irritants, trauma (including scratching), cold, scabies, and stasis to name a few.

These various forms of eczema will each be presented separately. As previously mentioned, the factor that characterize this group of skin disorders is their microvesicular changes. The keys to clinically differentiating eczematous skin diseases include inflammation, epithelial disruption, poor margination and lichenification. Papulosquamous skin diseases can look a lot like eczema, but the former group of skin diseases do not present with these four findings.

Inflammation is seen as redness, warmth, edema and tenderness. Usually, papulosquamous diseases are not so inflammatory in appearance. *Epithelial disruption* includes weeping, crusting, erosions, excoriation, and fissures. Rarely do papulosquamous diseases show any form of epithelial disruption. Eczematous diseases have diffuse borders and *poor margination* as compared to papulosquamous diseases and their sharp, well defined edges. *Lichenification* is thickening of the skin with formation of lichen-like scale due to chronic rubbing. Although papulosquamous disorders can be scaly, they are almost never lichenified. Thus, inflammation, epithelial disruption, poor margination, and lichenification are the four distinguishing clinical features of eczema.

The rest of this chapter will approach each type of eczema as a separate skin disease. The forms of eczema that will be discussed include: allergic contact dermatitis, irritant contact dermatitis, dyshidrosis, atopic dermatitis, stasis dermatitis, seborrheic dermatitis, and scabies. Although these skin diseases are all forms of eczema, their clinical presentations and treatments differ and, thus, should each be discussed separately.

▶ ALLERGIC CONTACT DERMATITIS

BACKGROUND

Allergic contact dermatitis (ACD) is an eczematous rash which erupts due to the skin's contact with a substance to which the patient has been previously sensitized. Thus, ACD is a T-cell mediated delayed—hypersensitivity reaction with a period of days to years between the initial contact to an allergen and the re-exposure which leads to the typical skin changes. This is a difficult problem. A systemic hypersensitivity can develop, when the exposure to antigen is extensive.

The delayed—hypersensitivity reaction seen in ACD is a type of immunologic event (type IV cell mediated) which begins with the initial skin contact with a substance called a hapten. This hapten binds to a protein in the epidermal cells and triggers a series of immunological steps. These steps lead to the production of antigen specific T-lymphocytes which are then ready to "attack" when the skin is next exposed to the original inciting agent. If such recontact occurs, the antigen specific T-lymphocytes migrate to the skin's surface, attach to the antigen, and cause the eczematous changes typical of ACD.

The skin changes occur approximately 48 hours after recontact with the inciting "allergen." The disease is self limited and resolves spontaneously within 10 to 20 days after removal of the causative factor. The symptoms as described below often lead an affected individual to seek treatment before the rash spontaneously resolves. If the etiologic hapten is not removed from contact with the skin, the rash may become chronic or might worsen. The skin's sensitization to a substance remains for many years after the initial insult, but slowly decreases with time if the hapten does not come in contact with the skin.

It is not known why certain substances often lead to contact dermatitis while others do not cause skin changes. Ninety percent of all allergic contact dermatitis is caused by poison ivy/oak/sumac, nickel, formaldehyde, paraphenylediamine (a black dye), neomycin, benzocaine, parabens (a preservative), chromate (used in shoes and cement), epoxy resins, fragrances, permanent wave solutions, and antioxidants (used in the rubber industry).

Poison ivy type contact dermatitis is the most common form of ACD. The antigen responsible for the skin's reaction is a pentadecatachol and is found in the plant's resin. It is an extremely potent antigen, and almost all individuals are sensitized if exposed. Jewelry induced ACD is due to its nickel content and is seen in approximately 20% of people who wear pierced—ring—jewelry and 2% of those individuals with other nonpierced forms of jewelry. Finally, the topical creams neomycin and benedryl are common allergens. It is important to note that topical *creams* are more likely to be allergenic than are topical *ointments.*

IN THE CLINIC

Individual lesions include erythematous, edematous papules and plaques. Weeping and crusting is evident if the eruption is acute. These skin changes give way to lichenification and fissuring as the disease becomes more chronic in duration. Blistering can be present and is most commonly seen in a poison ivy type etiology. Pruritus is quite common, although not universal, and can lead to subsequent excoriation from scratching.

The pattern of each group of lesions, as well as the overall body distribution and configuration, are important clues in diagnosing the underlying allergen. Grouping of lesions in linear patterns or as plaques with distinctive shapes and locations are almost pathognomonic for allergic contact dermatitis. For example, eyelid location with make-up allergen, linear arrangements with poison ivy type allergens, and the "earlobe sign" of a nickel allergy.

It is important to note that poison ivy type allergens can cause lesions on unexposed skin due to penetration of wet clothing and transfer of the antigenic resin via the hands. Also, dog fur can carry poison ivy oil which may be rubbed off on human skin and when burned or mulched, the plant's resin can carry on the wind or smoke. This air transfer phenomena can lead to extensive involvement of the face and other exposed areas. The resin can remain viable on firewood or pet fur for a significant period of time and may lead to outbreaks distant from time of actual plant exposure. Thus, a thorough history is often helpful in determining a poison ivy type of etiology.

DIAGNOSIS AND TREATMENT

The location and appearance of lesions along with a supporting history often leads not only to the diagnosis of allergic contact dermatitis, but to the determination of the actual allergen responsible. A suspicious etiologic agent can be confirmed via patch testing. This process involves application of suspected allergen to any area of normal skin. A positive response will demonstrate an inflammatory response with erythema, edema, and vesiculation. Although patch testing is a valuable diagnostic aid, it is rarely necessary if a thorough history and examination is performed. Reserve such tests for those individuals with severe skin changes whose etiology is difficult to otherwise determine.

Treatment begins with immediate removal of the allergen in question with further avoidance of contact with that agent. Open-to-air wet dressings of Burrow's solution or cool tap water three to four times each day, is quite helpful. An astringent lotion which contains camphor or menthol may be used on an as needed basis for mild pruritus. More significant itching will benefit from systemic antihistamines, for example, Atarax 25–50 mg every eight hours. Mid-potency topical steroids are often helpful if applied 3–4 times each day. Attempt to minimize the use of systemic steroids to only severe cases of allergic contact dermatitis, such as involvement of greater than 30% of the body surface area, genital lesions, or facial involvement. Be certain to taper steroids appropriately.

MANAGEMENT

To Manage

▼ Keep almost all cases
▼ Determine allergen if possible
▼ Remove allergen promptly
▼ Patient education in regards to cause of skin lesions and avoidance of etiologic agent
▼ Treat with:
  1. Open-to-air wet dressings of cool tap water or Burrow's solution
  2. Astringent lotion with camphor or menthol PRN mild pruritus
  3. Oral antihistamine (Adheres 25–50 mg every 8 hours) as needed for moderate to severe pruritus
  4. Topical mid-potency steroid TID-QID
  5. Oral corticosteroids if involvement of >30% of body surface area, genital lesions, or facial involvement.

Send

▼ All disseminated cases
▼ If bulla are present

▼ If patch testing is necessary

▼ Severe cases that do not respond to above treatments in 5 days

PROGNOSIS

ACD has an excellent prognosis as long as the etiologic agent is removed from the patients environment. As previously mentioned, ACD may become chronic in nature if the inciting agent is kept in contact with the patient's skin. Chronic eczema and its treatment will be dealt with specifically later in this chapter.

▶ IRRITANT CONTACT DERMATITIS

BACKGROUND

Irritant contact dermatitis is a common skin problem seen by most family practitioners. It can almost always be treated in the primary care setting with only rare need for consultation and never a need to refer. Unlike allergic contact dermatitis, this eczematous disease is not immunologic. Rather, irritant contact dermatitis arises when the outermost layers of skin are affected primarily by an environmental insult. Allergy is not involved.

Irritant contact dermatitis arises in two different skin models. Either a contacting substance leads to injury with overdrying (xerosis) of the skin or to excessive moisture entrapment (maceration). An example of the xerotic form of irritant contact dermatitis is exposure of hand skin to a solvent. The solvent damages the skin directly and leads to an overdry environment. Repeated exposure to something as simple as hand soap can cause xerotic ICD. An example of the macerated form of ICD is diaper dermatitis or diaper rash. Almost all diaper rash is ICD. A wet diaper is left in contact with the skin for a prolonged period of time which causes damage to the skin's epithelium and the formation of ICD Candida may become involved secondarily and further worsen the skin disease.

IN THE CLINIC

The clinical presentation of ICD depends on the source of the irritation which leads to the typical skin findings. ICD requires a sufficiently insulting irritant, thus , a thorough history will usually provide the source without need for further investigations. Ask the patient about exposure to chemicals, change in laundry detergents, and such. Two types of skin findings can be present in ICD—xerosis and maceration.

First, consider the xerotic type of ICD. The lesions consist of poorly marginated patches or plaques with associated erythema, pain, scale, erosion, fissuring, and lichenification. The stronger or the more prolonged the exposure to the irritant, the worse the inflammation present. Pruritus often occurs, but it is mild with rare excoriation. Weeping and crusting are also uncommon in the xerotic form of ICD.

The macerated variety of ICD occurs when skin is exposed to a moisture laden environment for a prolonged period of time. Such conditions include sweaty feet, wet diapers, wet body folds and wet hand work to name a few. Such environments will lead to fluid entrapment against the skin with subsequent overhydration and maceration. When the intertriginous areas are involved and there is *no* overlying skin disruption, the disease is called intertrigo. But, if epithelial damage is associated with the wet intertriginous area, the disease is considered ICD.

DIAGNOSIS AND TREATMENT

The diagnosis of irritant contact dermatitis is purely clinical. A thorough day-to-day history and physical exam is all that is necessary to delineate ICD from other forms of eczema. Since this disease is not allergen mediated, patch testing is of no value.

Thorough history taking may be vital in diagnosing some manageable causative factors from a complex list of possible offending agents. Once determined, removal of all offending agent from contact with the skin's surface is the mainstay of treatment and is essential for resolution of the skin rash. Rigid work circumstances often lead to difficulty removing the offending substance from the patient's environment. In such cases, protection and patient education are key components of therapy. Large, non-restrictive rubber gloves *with cotton liners* should always be employed under these circumstances. Also, maceration may be avoided by frequent changing of sweaty socks, wet gloves, and soggy diapers. Those with ICD of the hands should decrease the use of soap and water as much as possible.

In addition to these preventative measures, the skin must be thoroughly lubricated at least twice daily. Follow the guidelines under management in regards to how much lubricant should be employed in order to ensure efficacy.

MANAGEMENT

To Manage

- ▼ Plan to treat all cases in the primary care setting
- ▼ Patient education
- ▼ Avoid contact with offending irritant
- ▼ Decrease use of soap and hot water—use bath oil or Cetaphil as a substitute for soap.
- ▼ Pat skin dry rather than rub dry
- ▼ If maceration is involved, avoid allowing wet materials to be in contact with the skin for prolonged time periods without interval for drying.
- ▼ Lubricate with cream rather than lotion (Eucerin, Cetaphil, etc.)
- ▼ Apply approximately:

    1 tablespoon for each arm

    1 tablespoon for each leg

    2 tablespoons for each thigh

    2 tablespoons for trunk

    1 tablespoon for each hand/foot
- ▼ You know you have used enough cream if it takes about 5 minutes to rub the substance into the skin.
- ▼ Barriers such as rubber gloves may be used with the lubrication to improve response to therapy.

Send

Referral is not necessary if patient truly has ICD. Refer if patient isn't improving.

PROGNOSIS

Excellent if above steps employed. If the treatment does not improve the skin within 3–5 days, then the diagnosis of ICD should be suspect. Complications to ICD are quite rare.

▶ ATOPIC DERMATITIS

BACKGROUND

This autosomal dominantly inherited disorder leads to immunologic changes that cause the epithelial disruption and the itch/scratch cycle. Exactly how this immune event occurs is not known, but for some reason, it leads these individuals to scratch otherwise normal appearing skin leading to the commonly seen rash of atopic dermatitis. Precipitating factors include psychologic stressors, wet/moist skin conditions, and overdry skin conditions.

These irritation factors cause nerve endings in the skin to become excited and lead to scratching. A hallmark of atopic dermatitis is the patient's inability to control the itch/scratch cycle which leads to further skin changes typical of atopic dermatitis. The scratching further irritates nerve endings, which causes more itching which leads to more scratching, etc. Obtaining a thorough history that includes this itching is important in diagnosing this disease.

Individuals with atopic dermatitis also usually possess other "atopic" features such as allergic rhinitis, asthma, elevated IgE antibodies, dermatographism, xerosis, or keratosis pilaris. Although a patient may have other features of "atopy" they may present with the skin changes alone. Also, many individuals with atopic dermatitis also have a family history of "atopy" as above.

IN THE CLINIC

The rash presents as a poorly marginated set of erythematous plaques and patches in areas exposed to wet environments—groin, occiput, feet, antecubital fossa, popliteal fossa, and buttocks and cheeks in infants—and overdry environments—hands, dorsal feet, lower legs, etc. Scale is minimal.

A hallmark is the large degree of excoriation that is present and the patient's history of frequent itching and scratching. The presence of actual lichenification from chronic rubbing is indicative of a more chronic form of atopic dermatitis.

Also, as the physician, you should obtain a thorough history and a pertinent physical examination to rule out the presence of other "atopic" features.

DIAGNOSIS AND TREATMENT

The diagnosis of atopic dermatitis is purely clinical. Usually, the presence of excoriation and the history of frequent and persistent itching/scratching is useful in making the correct diagnosis.

When treating atopic dermatitis, patients need to be informed of the chronic nature of this skin disease and its waxing and waning features. They must learn that exacerbations are caused by wet or over dry environments as well as psychological stress and therefore, individuals must learn to adapt their lifestyles to minimize outbreaks of these skin lesions. Check for scabies.

Scratching should be reduced as soon as possible during an acute outbreak. This step is best accomplished via topical mid-potency steroids with heavy lubrication twice each day until rash improves, then once each day until resolves. Steroid creams may be combined with wet soaks of Burrow's solution up to three times daily. In very chronic patches, ointments. If the pruritus is severe, one might consider adding oral antihistamines such as Atarax 25–50 mg three times each day. Although oral steroids may be incorporated, they are rarely necessary, unless the skin changes are severe and the rash fails to respond to more conservative treatment as outlined above. If all the above regimens fail, the patient should be referred to a dermatologist to confirm the suspected diagnosis and attempt more complicated, time consuming therapies such as tar treatments and PUVA light therapy.

Once an outbreak is resolved, a patient with atopic dermatitis must be religious about frequent (3–4 times a day) lubrication and avoidance of stressors, increased relaxation, and should take care to not allow their skin to be exposed to over drying or to maceration. Again, patient education of the above is key. No simplistic treatment will succeed.

MANAGEMENT

To Manage

▼ Keep all cases unless not responsive to below therapy in 2 weeks time.

▼ Frequent—3–4 times—soaks with cool tap water or Burow's solution to reduce pruritus

▼ Mid-potency steroid cream (1% on face/genitals) twice each day until rash improves, then once a day until resolves

▼ Antihistamines such as Atarax 25–50 mg up to 3 times each day as needed for pruritus

▼ Oral steroids in short burst/taper in addition to above if case is severe or unremittable. Watch for exacerbation of rash once oral steroids are tapered off

▼ Patients must be educated

1. Frequent lubrication with sufficient cream/ointment 3–4 times daily between outbreaks. See section on irritant contact dermatitis management (pg.) for amount of lubricant that should be employed.
2. Avoid all xerotic environments—example—frequent hand washing with soap and water, hot showers, etc.
3. Avoid wet environments—example—wet diapers, sweaty socks, helmet/hat use, etc.
4. Avoid psychological stress and increase relaxation techniques.

PROGNOSIS

Unfortunately, atopic dermatitis is a chronic, waxing and waning disease for life. But, patient education as above is key. If an individual can keep their skin lubricated, avoid stressors and irritants, they will have a much greater chance of tight control then if these preventative measures are overlooked.

 SCABIES

BACKGROUND

Another eczematous skin condition arises as a result of cutaneous infestation by a mite, sarcoptes scabies. These mites are tiny, only about one-third a millimeter in diameter, and are difficult to visualize with the naked eye. Infestation is seen most often in children and adolescents. Although adults may have this mite on their body, they often do not demonstrate the rash, due to a fully developed immune system. Thus, though adults and children will both be infested, only the younger individuals usually present with skin changes and pruritus. This concept is important when treating the disease as will be described later.

Scabies is always spread via skin to skin contact and is often spread sexually. Poverty and overcrowded living conditions are other risk factors. Convincing studies demonstrate that the disease is not transmitted via fomites such as bed liners and clothing as was previously thought. The disease is very pruritic and it progresses in an individual via scratching which is difficult to control.

IN THE CLINIC

The scabies mite burrows into the superficial layers of the skin leaving behind a flesh-colored ridge. These burrows are about $^1/_2$ to 1 cm. In length and only 1 mm in diameter. If a burrow is scraped and examined microscopically, one may visualize the ova, feces, or possibly even an intact mite. Unfortunately, the severe pruritus that the infestation causes leads to scratching of these burrows and it is often difficult to find the intact burrows. Scratching leads to the typical eczematous lesions—erythematous, poorly marginated papules and plaques with crusting and excoriation.

The lesions are usually seen on the scalp, wrists, ankles, web spaces of finger and toes, nipples, umbilicus, and the genitals. As the disease becomes more chronic in nature, the lesions will be more widespread and are often seen on the trunk, arms, and legs.

If a patient presents with the above typical skin changes, then the patient should be carefully examined for intact burrows. If such a burrow is found, a thin shave of the burrow roof should be microscopically examined along with material scraped from the base of the lesion. The scraped material should be examined under low power in immersion oil and with a coverslip in place. Practice of this technique leads to improved yield of ova, feces, and mites. Any patient with suspected scabies should be looked over thoroughly for burrows and scraped accordingly. If mites or ova are found, the diagnosis has been made quickly, efficiently, and at low cost to the patient. Unfortunately, it takes time to perfect scraping techniques. So, if the disease is suspected with a corroborating history, treatment should be initiated even in the absence of burrows and/or positive scrapings.

DIAGNOSIS AND MANAGEMENT

Identification of mites, feces, or ova is a bit difficult and requires a properly performed scrape. Even if performed properly, the scrape is successful in only about half of the attempts made. Identification is helpful, but characteristic lesions, especially with history of exposure, are all that is necessary to treat. The value of the scraping is that it justifies an elaborate effort in treating many family members, some of whom are most uncooperative and unwilling to believe they are probably personally infested.

A scrape consists of:

1. Trying to find an intact burrow on a cluster of new papules without much damage from excoriation.
2. Lifting off the roof of the burrow with a scalpel.
3. Scraping the base of the burrow with the scalpel.
4. Viewing the specimen on a slide under low power microscopy in mineral oil.
5. Finding characteristic mites, ova, or feces.

Management of scabies involves reducing the pruritus and eliminating the mites and ova. Itching is improved with the use of antihistamines, such as Atarax, at doses of 25 to 50 mg every eight hours. Topical Synalar may also be employed to aid in the reduction of pruritus. If the itching is severe, a Prednisone taper can be employed.

Topical Lindane 1% cream or lotion may be used in nonpregnant adults to rid the skin of ova and mites. It must be applied to all contacts and should be used over the entire skin surface from the neck down. Leave the Lindane in place for 4–6 hours before rinsing. Repeat this procedure in 1 week to ensure elimination of all ova.

Elimite may be safer than Lindane in children and pregnant women. It is applied to the entire skin surface for 6 hours as is Lindane, but treatment may be repeated in 24 hours to ensure efficacy.

MANAGEMENT

To Manage

▼ Keep all acute cases:
   1. Reduce pruritus with antihistamines (Atarax 25–50 mg every 8 hours) and/or topical Synalar (fluocinolone acetonicle 0.025%) BID for 2 weeks. May need oral Prednisone for severe pruritus— (40 mg/d with taper over 7 days.)
   2. Eliminate mites and ova with topical ointments—treat *ALL* contacts.

  a. Nonpregnant adults: Lindane (Kwell) 1% cream or lotion to *entire* skin surface from neck down to toes. Leave on at least 6 hours and then rinse thoroughly with water. Reapply after one week to eliminate all ova.
  b. Elimite is as effective as Lindane but safer in children <1 year old and pregnant women. Apply from neck down to toes. Leave on for 24 hours. Then reapply another layer and wait additional 24 hours before washing with soap and water.

▼ Bed linens, clothing need *not* be specially handled.

▼ Treat all family members at the same time.

Send

Those patients with chronic eczemas that do not respond to therapy (atopic dermatitis-type). Phototherapy is often helpful in these individuals.

PROGNOSIS

The lesions seen in scabies usually resolve in 7–14 days after treatment is initiated. The pruritus caused by the mite actually improves sooner—often within 24–72 hours of therapy. Treatment of scabies is extremely effective if the above therapy specifics are closely followed. The major source of failure arises from reinfection by untreated contacts. Thus, be certain to emphasize the treatment of all frequent skin-to-skin contacts—even if they belong to another household.

If a scabies infestation was severe, a form of chronic eczema may persist after all the mites have been eliminated. Do not continue to repeat scabicide treatment because Lindane may cause further irritant dermatitis in these patients. Treat these chronic eczema patients as you would an individual with atopic dermatitis (refer to specific section). If this therapy is not effective within 2 weeks of initiation then referral to a dermatologist for phototherapy is often useful.

▶ STASIS DERMATITIS

BACKGROUND

This form of eczema is found in those patients who develop chronic venous stasis, actually, persisting edema of the lower extremities.

The constant edema causes the skin to stretch and itch. The patient responds by scratching and the itch/scratch cycle ensues. Patients with varicose veins as the etiology of their lower extremity stasis are commonly affected due to the chronicity of the swelling.

IN THE CLINIC

Stasis dermatitis presents as red to red-purple scaling plaques with poor demarcation and overlying excoriation. Weeping, crusting, and fissuring are commonly seen as well. These changes begin around the ankles and as the disease progresses, the rash may spread both proximally and distally. The skin changes may become severe if stasis continues and treatment is not initiated. Severe stasis dermatitis demonstrates ulcer formation. Stasis ulcers are typically 1–5 cm erythematous, painful lesions associated with stasis dermatitis. If the stasis dermatitis is chronic, often brownish, hyperpigmented plaques on the ankles and lower legs are seen between acute dermatitis flares. Consider diabetes.

DIAGNOSIS AND TREATMENT

Stasis dermatitis is purely a clinical diagnosis. The typical skin changes as outlined above, when associated with chronic edema of the lower extremities, is difficult to misdiagnose.

Treatment consists of removing all crusts with Burow's wet dressing three times each day. Topical, mid-potency steroids twice a day are often beneficial as well. Severe cases benefit from Unna boot therapy with weekly dressing changes. Remember, the skin changes will reoccur if the edema is not resolved. Thus, compression stockings and elevation are important additions to long term management of this disease.

MANAGEMENT

To Manage

▼ Keep most cases
▼ Evaluation and compression stockings
▼ Burow's solution 3 times each day
▼ Topical mid-potency corticosteroids twice each day
▼ May require Unna boot therapy with weekly dressing changes

▼ Ulcerations—above, plus wet to dry dressings if necessary. Watch for secondary bacterial infection

▼ Prevention—minimize edema via prophylactic use of compression stockings, elevation of extremities, and surgery if candidate (varicose veins), chronic lymphedema pumps daily if necessary

Send

▼ Cases that require Unna boots if unfamiliar with their use

▼ Stasis ulcerations that fail to heal or enlarge.

▼ Cases that do not respond to management as outlined above.

PROGNOSIS

The patient should be warned that as long as edema is present, the stasis dermatitis will reoccur. All efforts should be made to resolve the edema in addition to treating the skin manifestations.

CASE STUDY

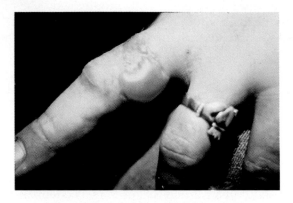

S: An 18 year old white female presents to your clinic in Seattle. She complains of a 6–7 day history of an itchy red lesion on her abdomen and right middle finger. The young women is a musician by profession. Her preferred instrument being the drums. The patient states she has just moved to the city from her home town of Pawhuska, Oklahoma because she heard the opportunity for musicians was great in Seattle (and not too hot in Oklahoma). She auditioned and secured a job with an all-female band as their new drummer. Apparently, one of the bands trademarks is multiple areas of body piercing and there has been pressure from the other band members for her to follow their lead. She admits to having her navel pierced about 2 weeks prior at a downtown tattoo parlor. Also, wears an Irish "clatter" ring. She has kept the same silver colored ring in since the day of piercing as instructed despite the increased redness and itching. She denies any fever, chills or other complaints. Otherwise has been feeling well.

O: Pleasant young female who appears slightly underweight but otherwise healthy.

HEENT: Wir skin of ears pierced x2 cm right and x5 on left. All holes filled with either gold hoops or studs. Each of the pierced sites is inflammed.
SKIN: Above HEENT
—There is a 1cm x 2.5cm patch of poorly marginated scaling erythema surrounding the patients navel. Puncture wound with platinum

colored stud earing present at approximately the center of this patch in the navel itself. Weeping, crusting with generalized vesiculation is present as well. Excoriation and edema moderate. Mildly warm to palpation but nontender. No exudate is noted.
—Otherwise WNL
Rest of examination including inguinal/axillary lymph nodes and abdomen are WNL.

A: Allergic Contact Dermatitis—probable nickel of navel

P: The jewelry was removed from the navel immediately. Advised patient probably allergic to nickel. She admits all the earrings in her ears are 18 karat gold and she never removes or changes these pieces of jewelry.

Advised patient to avoid any nickel jewelry in the future, including the "gold" earrings.

Treated the lesion with open-to-air—dressing with cool tap water every 4–6 hours to aid in removing crusts and improving pruritus. Prescribed a topical midpotency steroid to rub into affected area twice each day for about 2 weeks. She was instructed she could use an oral OTC antihistamine if above not enough to improve the itching. If the rash should not improve within 2 weeks or worsen, she was to return for reevaluation and possible referral for patch testing.

NOTE: *All gold jewelry has a nickel content. Pure gold is not used as jewelry.*

PATIENT EDUCATION HANDOUT
ECZEMA

Your rash is a type of skin disease called eczema in general. The specific type of eczema you have is called

_____.

Your doctor has given you instructions on decreasing the itching of your skin. Follow his/her instructions as follows:

_____

_____

_____

If the doctor has prescribed a steroid cream for your skin, use it only as often and in the areas he/she has instructed as follows:

_____

_____

_____

_____

Keep your skin well lubricated/moisturized. Do this by using a cream or ointment rather than a lotion. We recommend

_____.

Use *lots* of moisturizer—it should take 5 minutes to rub it all in. Use the moisturizer at least 2 times a day—especially after bathing.

Avoid exposing your skin to water unless necessary.

Take showers with warm (not *hot*) water and try not to shower > 1 time each day unless necessary.

Avoid harsh-deodorant type-soaps. The type of soap/cleanser recommended is

_____.

Pat—don't rub—your skin dry.

Do not keep wet clothes/socks on for any long time—change these often if wet/sweaty.

Other instructions:

_____

_____

_____

Call if any questions, concerns, or if no improvement.

▶ HERPES SIMPLEX

BACKGROUND

Herpes virus hominus is a DNA virus with two distinct definable strains—HSV1 and HSV2. The herpes virus can cause cutaneous infections of the lips and the genital skin. These are termed herpes labialis and herpes genitalis respectively.

Recurrent herpes labialis is usually caused by HSV1, but can be caused by HSV2. It is usually an infection of young adults and can be transmitted via skin-skin or skin-mucosa contact. There exists an approximate incubation period that ranges from 2 days to 3 weeks. This virus can lay dormant between episodes of skin lesion manifestation. Recurrences of herpes labialis may be triggered by stress, concomitant illness, dental care or UV radiation. The initial infection may be undistinguishable, clinically, from a viral pharyngitis, usually in childhood. Herpes genitalis is also a sexually transmitted skin disease due to infection by the herpes virus hominus. But the genital form of herpes simplex is usually due to HSV2, but HSV1 can also cause identical lesions. Transmission is through direct skin-skin contact with an infected individuals and its incubation period is the same as that for herpes labialis—2 days to 3 weeks.

Herpes simplex infections on the lip may occur as a result of direct trauma, dental care, sunburn, irritants in food and menstrual cycle influences.

Each episode of herpes simplex genitalis lesions lasts 7–14 days and contagion to susceptible sexual partners is possible during the first 5 days. About $^1/_2$ of all patients will experience 1 or more recurrences without being reinfected. These recurrences are best thought of as re-outbreaks. Recurrences are always less severe than the first episode. These recurrences are due to the virus's tendency to proceed into a latent phase in the dorsal root ganglion between outbreaks. The virus remains latent until conditions lead to a re-outbreak. Such conditions include: trauma during intercourse, menses, vaginal infections, and stress. These "fatigue factors" trigger the virus to move from the dorsal root ganglia, out to the skin via the sensory nerve roots. Here, the virus quickly replicates and leads to the formation of the typical vesicular lesions. Seventy percent of all people harbor one or both types of herpes virus through their entire lives, although many will never experience a single outbreak of the lesions.

As previously noted, both HSV1 and 2 can show venereal spread. Although the majority of sexual spread occurs while lesions are present, some viral shedding can occur during the asymptomatic latent phase. Thus, the appearance of the lesions can occur due to exposure to a clinically infected individual 3–5 days before, exposure to an asymptomatic viral shedding 3–5 days before, or activation of a latent infection that was acquired earlier, but never had an initial outbreak.

IN THE CLINIC

Herpes labialis and genitalis can be primary, but is typically recurrent in nature. Primary herpes infection is characterized by skin lesions which appear as clustered groups of 3–8 vesicles on an erythematous—plaque-like base. Each vesicle is usually 1–3 mm in diameter. The vesicle roof is friable and will often erode, leaving a shallow erosion. These erosions may be associated with a yellow crust. These skin changes are almost always accompanied by regional lymphadenopathy and may have associated headache, fever, and fatigue. The skin changes usually fully heal in 2–4 weeks without scarring.

Recurrent herpes simplex is characterized by a prodromal phase 1–2 days before the eruption of skin lesions. This prodrome varies from localized itching to pain to burning. There are usually no associated systemic symptoms. The skin lesions are identical to those in the primary form of herpes labialis—but much smaller. The skin changes are often associated with striking lymphadenopathy. These lesions heal faster with full resolution in 1–2 weeks. Again, scarring is usually not present. The importance of the prodromal phase becomes apparent when we discuss treatment.

Herpes labialis lesions may occur on any mucosal surface. Usually they are seen periordally, on the lips, cheek, nose, or distal finger (known as herpetic whitlow). Wrestlers commonly have outbreaks on their neck, shoulders and head due to traumatic contact during competition. Transfer of the herpes virus, to the cornea is of great concern in these athletes as well as those who participate in boxing and football. Thus, participation in these sports should be limited or fully avoided when active herpes labialis is present so as to prevent possible corneal involvement.

Herpes genitalis is most commonly seen in males on the penile shaft, glans, prepuce, scrotum and buttocks. All recurrent herpes genitalis in men is on the penile shaft. In females, infections can be on the labia, perineum, breasts or thighs. Most recurrent herpes genitalis in females is on the labia.

In addition, the family physician must also be aware of the possibility of infection in the neonate born to a woman with a herpes simplex infection at or just prior to delivery. Although an infected infant may have skin lesions, many will develop systemic herpes infections without signs of cutaneous disease. When herpes simplex is systemic in a neonate, the disease is severe and can be fatal. Treatment of the infected neonate is via Acyclovir 30 mg/kg/d intravenously, or an equivalent therapy. Physicians should follow the protocol for their obstetrical unit in regards to how to manage a pregnant female with active herpes lesions. Special care is extremely important when she has a cluster of acute herpes genitalis lesions present.

DIAGNOSIS AND TREATMENT

Almost all cases of herpes simplex—either labialis or genitalis—can be easily diagnosed clinically. If the lesions are in question a *Tzanck Smear* can be performed. This test involves removing the fluid from an intact vesicle and placing it on a slide. After drying, Wright's or Gremsa's stain is applied and it is viewed microscopically. If one sees multinucleated giant Keratinocytes or accinthocytes, then a herpes virus infection is present. Another diagnostic option is the 48 hour *Viral Culture*. One cultures fluid from the vesicle or the floor of an erosion. But, most herpes infections are easily diagnosed clinically.

Treatment of acute herpes labialis and genitalis is identical. Local modalities including frequent warm soaks are very beneficial. Unfortunately topical Acyclovir has not been shown to be effective. If the patient is seen during the prodromal phase, or within the first 24 hours after the lesions erupt, they may be treated with an oral antiviral agent. Both Acyclovir and Valcyclovir have been demonstrated to have equally efficacious results if used early as described above. Acyclovir is given as 200 mg, 5 times each day for 5 days. Valcyclovir is 500mg, 2 times a day for 10 days. The cost of these two drugs is equivalent. Acyclovir has been given prophylactically to some patients as 200 mg, 3 times a day or 400 mg twice a day. Patients may remain on this dose for up to one year. Remember herpes ZOSTER is treated in a higher dose, preferably with Valcyclovir.

MANAGEMENT

To Manage

- ▼ Keep most cases
- ▼ Culture only those lesions that are atypical
- ▼ Local modalities—warm soaks twice a day to prn.
- ▼ If caught within 24 hours of lesion outbreak:
  Acyclovir 200mg—5 times a day for 5 days *or*
  Valcyclovir 500mg—twice daily for 10 days
- ▼ If history of frequent outbreaks: Prophylactic Acyclovir at 200 mg, 3 times a day
  or 400mg twice a day.
- ▼ Prevention in contact sports—required patient education
- ▼ Symptomatic treatment of fatigue, fever, stress, sunburn and trauma to prevent recurrences.

Send

- ▼ Only if lesions do not respond to above treatment and diagnosis is in question.
- ▼ Or if persistent ulcerations or nodules after above treatment.
- ▼ Patients with wide spread or ulcerative disease—they are probably immunoincompetent.

PROGNOSIS

The recurrent outbreaks of herpes simplex virus get less severe with age. Patient with HIV or other immune system deficiencies may have widespread cutaneous changes or dissemination. Herpes can spread widely and dangerously into preexisting skin diseases, such as atopic eczema or intertrigo.

PEARLS AND PITFALLS

- ▼ Valcyclovir may be used prophylactically and it will decrease the recurrence rate to almost zero. But, once the medication is stopped, new outbreaks frequently do occur.

▾ HSV may spread to eye (especially in contact sports) with possible corneal scarring.

▾ May cause allergic reaction manifested as urticaria or erythema multiforme or even an exanthem.

▾ May cause a recurrent neuritis as does herpes zoster.

▾ Rarely causes deep scar or persistent nodule.

▾ May occasionally take a dermatomal pattern, mimicking zoster.

CASE STUDY

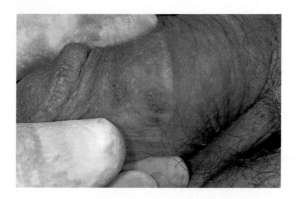

S: A 23 year old white male graduate student presents with a history of "breaking out" in a painful rash on his penis. He felt a burning sensation there 3 days ago. He states he first saw the blisters when he awoke today. He has had a similar rash about 2 years ago but it involved his thighs as well. He is currently dating 3 girls and has sex with all of them (on separate occasions). He never uses a condom because he doesn't "like the way they feel." He admits to being very stressed over the past 1 month due to trying to finish his thesis. He has a tender bump on his groin. He has no other complaints.

O: Skin—penile shaft demonstrated a 2cm erythematous erosion with a few small clustered vesicles at its inferior aspect. Extremely tender to touch. There is a 1 cm left injuncel lymph node. No penile discharge. The rest of the skin exam is normal.

A: Herpes Genitalis

P: 1. Warm soaks as needed
2. Acyclovir 200mg 5 times a day for 5 days or Valcyclovir 500mg 2 times a day for 10 days.
3. Patient education re: Herpes infections as sexually transmitted disease.
4. Recommend NO sexual intercourse at all while lesions are present. Use condoms regularly.
5. Test for further STDs while in clinic.

PATIENT EDUCATION HANDOUT
HERPES SIMPLEX

Herpes in the genital area is contagious and spread by sexual contact. You should limit your sexual behavior whenever open lesions are present. A condom is required.

You may feel a localized burning/pain/or itching in an area before skin lesions develop—this is normal for herpes.

If you desire oral medication that can prevent or shorten the time the lesions are present, see your doctor *immediately* when you have the burning/pain/ or itching or within 24 hours of the skin lesions first showing up.

You may use warm, wet soaks to areas as often as needed. These should help with pain, itching and will improve the appearance of the lesions.

Herpes can be inoculated into the eye from fingers. Wash your hands and be cautious.

▶ Moles (Nevi)

BACKGROUND

Nevi of the common melanotytic type, are small pigmented skin lesions that vary in color from flesh-tones to black. Flat nevi are termed *junctional* as regards their histopathologic pattern, while most elevated nevi are either *intradermal* or *compound*. All true nevi are benign processes that arise from naturally occurring melanocytes. These melanocytes rise up to the epidermis before birth after which they undergo an immense increase in number and disorganization of arrangement. This disorganized packed mass of previous melanocytic cells is then termed a nevus. The architecture of this unorganized packing is what determines the visual appearance of the nevus. For example, a sweat gland nevus is a clear and shiny papule composed of several hundred disorganized, tightly packed sweat glands just below the skin's surface. A connective tissue nevus has a palpable, cobblestone-like surface and is made up of numerous jumbled connective tissue cells. Thus, the whole variety of nevi is very large. The skin can display at least one kind of nevus for every different tissue in the skin.

Earlier, we described melanocytic nevi in regards to their overall height. A junctional nevus is flat and is composed of a disorganized pack of cells that is found at the dermal-epidermal junction. The raised nature of a compound nevus is derived from the jumbled cells sitting in the dermal-epidermal layer as well as the dermis itself. Finally, when the mass of nevus cells lies solely within the dermis, the resulting raised lesion is termed an intradermal nevus.

The occurrence and preponderance of nevi is inherited within families. In fact, not only are individuals likely to develop moles if their parents have moles, but the same nevi, with the same architecture and distribution may be seen regularly in several family members.

IN THE CLINIC

The majority of nevi first begin to appear at age two and arise in phases throughout life associated with growth. Thus, crops of new nevi may be seen at age two, six, eight, and at puberty. Very few new nevi will arise denovo after the teen years. Rarely, an infant is born with a nevus. These lesions are termed *congenital nevi*. Congenital nevi are usually light brown to black in color, greater than 5 cm in diameter, with rough, hairy pelt-like surface. Unlike other nevi, congenital variants may develop into malignant melanoma. Although this transformation occurs in only 1% of congenital nevi, the threat is significant enough that removal of some larger, more active nevi is suggested. The excision of these lesions need not occur in infancy, but should be carried out prior to puberty. Most small congenital nevi will require no treatment.

When nevi first develop, they are junctional in nature. In other words, new nevi are always flat. Then as the patient ages, the nevus will change in its height dimensions and substance progressing from junctional to compound to intradermal in appearance. Hair may develop over time as well. Thus, all moles should be expected to naturally "grow" in size, but the changes should be gradual and overall appearance should not be altered dramatically. Nevi will naturally undergo these minor height and substance changes until the mid-twenties. After this point in life, a nevus becomes more stable in its overall appearance, but slowly becomes more fibrous and pedunculate in the later years. Nevi are always changing.

The one exception to this rule is the pregnant female. Nevi will naturally darken in color during pregnancy. During pregnancy, the pituitary becomes more active in its secretion of hormones, including MSH (melanocyte stimulating hormone). This increase in MSH will lead to rapid darkening of moles over a short time period. Although, these lesions change rapidly in color, alarm is not necessary. The chances of a nevus developing into a malignant melanoma during pregnancy is no greater than in the general population.

So, one might ask, what is the chance a mole will develop into malignant melanoma? Actually, the chance is quite small, about 1 in 100,000. Only 10% of *all* malignant melanomas develop from preexisting moles, while 90% arise denovo. Unfortunately, there exists no effective method by which to determine which moles will transform into malignant melanoma. It was previously thought that "dysplastic" nevi—a diagnosis based on histologic appearance—had a greater tendency to form malignant melanoma. This belief is no longer thought to be valid. A patient must possess "Familial Dysplastic Nevi" in order to actually have a greater chance of malignant melanoma developing from a dysplastic nevus. Thus, if a patient has a dysplastic nevus without family history of dysplastic nevi or malignant melanoma, their chance of developing this cancer is the same as the general population—1 in 100,000. Thus, the routine biopsing of moles to rule out malignant melanoma is costly and unwarranted. It is much more efficient and a better practice to clinically screen moles on a regular basis for those that might have an increased risk of developing into malignant melanoma.

Remember, no more than 10% of all melanomas arise in any pre-existing brown nevus. Most arise from normal appearing skin. Thus, a nevus that has existed for years that undergoes a small change is much less likely to be a malignant melanoma than a new lesion that changes rapidly. It is important to inform your patients of their distinction, for they are more aware of an acute change due to their ability to visualize their skin on a regular basis. Although very few moles will require biopsy, in light of the morbidity and mortality from malignant melanoma, it is essential that an effort be made to precisely diagnose those that do.

Every seborrheic keratosis, wart, pilar keratosis, vascular lesion, or even a darkly pigmented insect bite can be imagined to be a melanoma. Nevi that develop and change rapidly, especially after the mid-twenties should be thought of as suspicious. Changes in the ABCD criteria of nevi as listed below are important to document. Before considering biopsy—at least 2 of these 5 criteria should occur.

ABCDT means: Asymmetry, Border, Color, Diameter, and Texture.

1. **ASYMMETRY:** Most benign nevi are nearly oval or round in shape and could be seen as two nearly matching "halves" if sliced down the center (ie, symmetrical). If the best two halves are grossly out of match and asymmetrical, then consider a biopsy. A quick change in symmetry usually denotes a change in size and border as well.

2. **BORDER:** Little new islands, buds, streaks, or pseudopods off the original border of a nevus is a reason to excise. Also, borders are usually sharp, and a new patch of "fuzzy edge," especially if soot-black, would be a concern.

3. **COLOR:** Melanomas usually are black as patent leather and/or mottled irregularly with some pitch black dots. Also, a quick change to white, blue or red components is a strong sign for melanoma. Often with color change comes a change in texture or a new surface irregularity. These changes are reason for biopsy.

4. **DIAMETER:** Substantial rapid change in size is a reason to biopsy. *Remember* that all during life nevi are *gradually* enlarging. In early adolescence, pregnancy, or during illness nevi

may seem to change more solely because they darken. Try to distinguish these small changes in size from moles with an acute, significant size change.

5. **TEXTURE:** Even if other features remain constant, a new lump or erosion in a mole prompts a consideration of biopsy. Everyday trauma causes most of these common changes, so consider re-examination in 7–10 days.

Again, two of these criteria usually should be met before a "mole" is biopsied. Judge the "level of concern" from the extent of the change. Merely 1 of these criteria is not usually sufficient for biopsy. The patient with a single change should be reassured and evaluated every six months for two years to watch for further changes. If two years pass without any further development of the ABCDT criteria a mole should be considered "stable." A good way to follow moles is via a map or diagram of each mole and its location in the patient's chart. A thorough skin check should be part of *every* routine health maintenance examination.

DIAGNOSIS AND TREATMENT

Thus, the diagnosis of a nevus is clearly clinical in nature. If a nevus does not fulfill any of the above ABCDT criteria simple yearly skin checks during health maintenance examination are sufficient as screening. If one criteria is present, then the mole in question should be rechecked every six months for two years, then again annually at health maintenance exams. If two of the five criteria are present, the lesion should be biopsied promptly in the primary care clinic. All suspicious moles should be excised via a punch biopsy. Routinely, a 5 mm punch should be employed and the procedure carried out under clean (not necessarily sterile) conditions.

How To Punch

1. Choose the lesion and prep the area
2. Inject 1% Lidocaine without epinephrine, slowly and shallowly around the lesion. This technique allow rapid onset of anesthesia and minimal distortion of the specimen. Be sure to obtain a good skin wheal. DO NOT use epinephrine with the lidocaine because epinephrine changes the vessels.
3. Take your non-biopsing hand and stretch the skin surrounding

the lesion in the direction in which you want the skin to fall back into an ellipse.

4. Position the punch exactly *VERTICAL* to the plane of the skin, apply even pressure and a quick clockwise—counter clockwise drilling motion. Continue this action until the bottom of the dermis is reached. You should have a plug that will be a good histopathologic.

5. Easily lift the plug up with a bit of fat attached to the base. DO NOT crush the plug with forceps. Handle it gently at the free edges. Snip the plug free and place it in formalin.

6. The wound should be slightly elliptical if #3 above was followed. Close the wound with two widely spaced 4-0 or 5-0 ethilon or nylon sutures. Take generous bites with the needle to control bleeding.

After biopsing in the primary care clinic send the specimen to pathology. Do not waiver: write "melanoma" on the biopsy request. Unfortunately, pathologists over diagnose melanoma, thus a phone consult with your dermatologist to review the histopathology to consult and confirm the pathologist's diagnosis.

Pathologists can not be expected reliably to bring to the diagnosis all the complexity of some cases, because they lack the clinical training and do not see the individual patients or examine the lesions or know of special circumstances. The biopsy is only one small laboratory test. The clinicians must take responsibility for the consultation with the pathologist and final analysis of the case. Routinely, this should be done case by case with your dermatologists, whether or not the patient is to be sent on. This is a prime opportunity for collaborative quality review. This review should be carried out without difficulty, if close cooperation and mutual understanding is established between the primary care physician and the dermatologist.

If the biopsy demonstrates malignant melanoma the patient should be referred promptly to the dermatologist for further management.

MANAGEMENT

To Manage

▼ Keep almost all patients
▼ Measure and chart routinely

▼ If two or more of ABCDT criteria, biopsy promptly with punch technique and phone consult with dermatologist to confer on histopathology
▼ Reassure and educate patients as necessary

Send

1. *Highly* suspicious lesions which need definite, prompt total excision.
2. Patients with family history or Familial Dysplastic Nevus Syndrome

PROGNOSIS

Only 1 of 100,000 nevi will transform into malignant melanoma. The rest are benign and of no significant consequence. Remember that dysplastic nevi are of significance only in the context of Familial Dysplastic Nevi Syndrome. Patients with this rare syndrome should be referred to a dermatologist.

PEARLS AND PITFALLS

▼ Nevi occur in crops at age 2, 6, 8, and puberty.
▼ Very few nevi arise after mid-twenties.
▼ Nevi change throughout life but slowly and minimally.
▼ Worry about those nevi that change rapidly after age twenty.
▼ Follow ABCDT criteria for biopsy and management.
▼ Follow punch biopsy rules.
▼ Never forget the importance of reassurance and patient education.
▼ All moles are expected to darken during pregnancy.

CASE STUDY

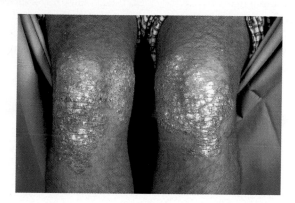

S: A 52 year old mailman presents to your clinic in rural southern Alabama with concern over a red, scaling plaques that he first noticed about 2 months prior but has been worsening since then. He states the rash is "kind of" itchy but more of a cosmetic problem than anything else. The rash began on his elbows and is now on his knees and buttocks as well. He is worried about what people think about the rash—especially since it is summer and he is wearing his shorts and short sleeved uniform while working. He denies any trauma, fever, chills, or other complaints. He was diagnosed 3 months previously with manic/depressive disorder for which he was placed on lithium. He is under the care of a psychiatrist for this illness. He is unaware if his lithium level has been checked recently. He states he has never had such a rash in the past, but remembers a paternal grandfather who had such red patches on his knees.

O: General—Pleasant middle aged male who appears his stated age. His affect is moderately blunted but he appears reliable. Vitals are stable. He is afebrile.

Skin: There are well demarcated, erythematous plaques present on the knees and elbows bilaterally and on his buttocks. The plaques are covered with moderately large scale. Peeling of a particularly large flake of skin on the right knee produces a tiny amount of bleeding. No evidence of excoriation is present.

—Rest of examination is not remarkable.

A: Psoriasis—classic form

P: 1. Lubricate, lubricate, lubricate (as per patient education handout and treatment section)

2. A topical midpotency steroid cream to be applied twice each day until rash improved, then decreased to once-a-day.
3. Serum lithium level to be checked. Lithium may aggrevate psoriasis.
4. Phone consultation with psychiatrist over possible association of psoriasis onset with lithium. Advise a change in medication for him manic/depressive disorder, if feasible.

PATIENT EDUCATION HANDOUT
PSORIASIS

Psoriasis is a skin disease you will have throughout life which will get better if you treat it correctly and may return if you do not.

Keep your skin well lubricated/moisturized. Do this by using a cream or ointment rather than a lotion. We recommend _____.

Use *lots* of moisturizer—it should take 5 minutes to rub it all in. Use the moisturizer at least 2 times a day—especially after bathing.

Avoid sunburn, injuries, and irritating substances which will make your disease worse.

Sunlight in small doses, without the threat of sunburn, can help your psoriasis.

Your doctor has prescribed _____.

Use this medication as follows:

_____
_____
_____

▶ Skin Cellulitis (Pyoderma)

BACKGROUND

The term cellulitis is often used in primary care settings to describe a bacterial skin infection when cellulitis can involve deeper layers such as muscle. A more appropriate label for bacterial infection only of the skin is "pyoderma." A pyoderma is an acute process that spreads through the dermal layers—often with an obvious site of bacterial entry. We live in a sea of bacteria, but only a few can cause pyoderma in immunologically intact individuals. By far, the two most common inciting agents are Staphylococcus aureus and Group A or B hemolytic Streptococcus (Strep pyogens). Often an infection will have manifestations of these two pathogens together.

All adults and children have many small pyodermas develop every month of their life. These may be manifested by bacterial invasion of small cuts, tinea lesions, insect bites, fissures, and excoriations. These are merely a few of the disturbances of intact epidermis that will invite colonization by the two bacteria previously mentioned. Luckily, most of these smaller processes heal on their own with the basics of "home" wound care.

Our concern is with those few infections that do not heal naturally and present in a varied spectrum in our clinical setting. No pathogenic bacteria will survive on wholly healthy, dry human skin. But, as above, even small injuries to the epidermis allow Staph/Strep to proliferate. If these wounds do not heal naturally and a sufficient number of bacteria are present, the lesions will spread via contiguous autoinoculation.

The majority of pyodermas involve the upper layers of the skin, but deeper layer and subcutaneous tissue may be involved if left untreated for a period of time. The key is early diagnosis with rapid initiation of appropriate antibiotics.

IN THE CLINIC

Pyoderma are characterized by erythematous, hot edematous plaques that are tender, restrict movement, and well demarcated from surrounding areas of skin. The size of the pyoderma will vary and they can spread in size quite rapidly. These plaques may demonstrate associated vesicles, bullae, erosions or central necrosis. The ac-

tual distribution of the skin change depends on the type of pyoderma, but almost all begin with an entry site and spread from there.
Below is further discussion of various forms of pyoderma.

Erysipelas is one of the few totally streptococcal pyodermas. It is
caused mainly by group A and occasionally by group C strep bacteria. It involves the lymphatics and spreads superficially. The plaques
are typical in their redness, edema, warmth, and good demarcation
but may be quite painful. Erysipelas often occurs on the face, beginning in or around the ear, and on the lower legs. It may easily resemble an allergic contact dermatitis, but there is usually more
edema and more pain. Overlying blisters may be present, and the local lymph nodes are reactive in erysipelas where they are not in
ACD. This pyoderma is easily treated as outlined below, but it can
actually be fatal if therapy is not initiated soon in the disease process.

Impetigo is a very superficial skin infection and typically demonstrates a mixed flora of Staph aureas and group A and B Hemolytic
Streptococcus. It usually affects children and adolescents and can be
caused by small areas of traumas to the skin that go without proper
wound care. Poor hygiene may be a contributing factor as well. The
plaques of impetigo begin as vesicles whose roofs break down, leaving shallow erosions with associated yellowish crusts. They may be
discrete or confluent in their distribution and are usually seen on the
face. Early impetigo may resemble herpes simplex labialis.

A form of impetigo appropriately termed *bullous impetigo* can occur. It is often seen in neonates and is rare in individuals over the age
of 12. The actual bulla are rarely visualized due to easy disruption of
the overlying roof and subsequent erosion formation. The most common sites of occurrence are the face, hands, elbows, and knees. A
variant of bullous impetigo is caused exclusively by staph aureas
and can lead to bullous "sheet-like" epidermal necrosis known as
Staphylococcus scalded skin syndrome. It is caused by a staph exotoxin
that disrupts epithelium and causes a clinical skin infection manifested as large pieces of peeling epithelium. Its "scalded-skin" comes
from its appearance which mimics a thermal burn. It, like bullous impetigo, is seen almost exclusively in children and usually begins in
the intertriginous areas.

A less common form of impetigo is ulcerative in nature and
termed *ecthyma*. Ecythema develop in skin lesions that have not been
treated well. They usually present as tender, red ulcers that may be
pruritic. The initial blister roof may be recalled by the patient, but is

so fragile it usually breaks down early in the disease process. This form of impetigo is seen predominately on the feet, ankles, legs, and thighs.

Toxic Shock Syndrome is another staphylococcal infection in which the skin breaks down due to toxin release. Blisters are not seen as in scalded skin syndrome. Rather, the skin lesions are erythematous plaques that may be widely scattered and have little crust, excoriations, or scale. They occur with associated fever, diarrhea, and hypotension in a systemic constellation of symptoms. The disease may be fatal and has been seen in women who use super-absorbent tampons during menstruation without frequent changing. Toxic Shock may occur with ordinary wound infections.

Folliculitis is a superficial skin infection caused by a mixture of staph aureas and group A B hemolytic streptococcus. The bacteria infect the hair follicle at its superficial level leading to erythematous pustules scattered over the skin. These lesions are rarely pruritic, but may be tender. Folliculitis is common on the face, scalp and legs. A variant is caused by pseudomonas aeruginosa and is termed "hot tub folliculitis" due to its presenting on the trunk and extremities of patients who recently used a hot tub.

A *furuncle* is a red, tender nodule that arose from a previous superficial folliculitis. These nodules are typically deep and warm to the touch, as well as quite painful to the inflicted individual. If multiple furuncles merge they can form a *carbuncle.* The distribution of furuncles and carbuncles is like that of folliculitis above.

Hidradenitis Suppurativa is a deep infection of the large apocrine-follicular structures. It is most commonly seen in the axilla and groin, but may be seen in the scalp or buttocks. It is chronic in nature and typified by large inflammatory nodules or abscesses which can be painful and may have associated purulent drainage. They are not associated with hair follicles and can lead to scarring.

Post-operative wound infections will usually appear 36 hours or more after surgery. They demonstrate the warmth, pain, erythema and edema associated with other pyoderma. Quick treatment is essential to prevent possible local and general spread of the bacteria.

Micrococci bacteremia is actually quite common with exercise, minor skin lesions, chewing, tooth cleaning, and coitus to name just a few. Only rarely does the immune-intact patient fail to clear the bacteremia with ease. If a patient's immune defenses are overridden, this full-blown septicemia can occur. Skin diseases are an important cause of septicemia which can be life-threatening. Thus, it is vital to treat bacterial skin infections early and correctly to prevent this possible negative outcome.

DIAGNOSIS AND TREATMENT

Pyoderma occur when the rich colony of common micrococci cause clinical infection. Over 99% of pyoderma are caused by staphylococcus aureas or streptococcus pyogenes and therapy needs to be aimed at eliminating these two bacteria. Thus, it is rarely cost-effective to perform a bacterial culture of a pyoderma. If you are questioning the diagnosis, for example—if delineating common atopic dermatitis from impetigo—a gram stain is the most cost-effective diagnostic approach. The gram stain should show the classic gram(+) cocci in pairs/clusters. If other bacteria predominate or if no significant bacteria are seen, then the diagnosis of pyoderma should be questioned.

If another etiology is suspected, based on gram stain, the appropriate culture should be performed. Look for dermatophytosis by the KOH examination. Tineas resemble pyodermas. Often a subsequent biopsy is needed to confirm the culture due to its poor sensitivity.

The treatment of pyoderma depends on their depth of invasion into the skin. The four mainstays of treatment are frequent cool soaks, topical bactroban twice daily, oral antibiotics 3–4 times daily, and appropriate incision and drainage, or even debridement.

Superficial involvement such as with folliculitis, impetigo, scalded skin syndrome, and ecthyma requires nothing more than cool, wet soaks every 2–3 hours to remove any overlying crust with topical bactroban applied twice each day.

Deeper infections such as furuncles, carbuncles, hidradenitis suppurativa, post operative wound infections, and erysipelas will require oral antibiotics. The most commonly employed is Cephalexin at doses of 500mg 3–4 times each day. These deep infections may also require incision, drainage, and possible packing to hasten recovery. If the patient has continued spread of the pyoderma despite oral antibiotics and ID where appropriate, then they will necessitate intravenous antibiotics. Usually Ancef at 1 gram every 8 hours until skin changes resolve will follow-up 10 day course of oral Keflex at 500mg 3 times each day with close out patient monitoring of the healing process.

MANAGEMENT

To Manage

▼ Keep most cases

▼ Cool soaks (possibly add Hebclens [antibacterial soap]) every 3–4 hours to clean off crust/overlying debris

▼ If superficial infection:

▼ Folliculitis

▼ Impetigo

▼ Ecthyma

▼ Scalded skin syndrome

   Use only topical bactroban twice daily—oral antibiotics are *not* necessary

▼ If deeper infection

   Furuncle/Carbuncle

   Hidradenitis suppurative

   Erysipelas

   Post-op wound infection

▼ Use oral Keflex 500mg 3–4 times a day for 7–10 days.

▼ If continued spread, then IV Ancef 1 gram every 8 hours with follow-up outpatient oral Keflex as above.

▼ TSS requires immediate IV antibiotics, but not steroids.

▼ Any nodule, cyst, or tract should be incised, drained, and packed as appropriate.

▼ Teach home wound care essential to all patients to prevent pyoderma/restrict their spread.

Send

▼ If elaborate skin surgery necessary (ex.: H. Supprativa with multiple tracts/apts.)

▼ Any necrotizing process

▼ Patients who are immune deficient and susceptible to frequent pyoderma.

PROGNOSIS

Prognosis is very good in almost all cases. About 5% of erysipelas is fatal and approximately 10% of patients with Toxic Shock Syndrome will die. Deep furuncles, carbuncles, and hidradenitis suppurativa may lead to scarring. Early and appropriate treatment should limit the scar.

PEARLS AND PITFALLS

▼ Allergic contact dermatitis, tinea, and Herpes Simplex infections can mimic early pyoderma.

▼ Immune compromised patients (including diabetics) are prone to pyoderma. Prompt treatment is essential.

▼ A patient with recurrent pyoderma may benefit from bactroban to nares twice a day for 5 days as prophylactic measure.

▼ Removing crusts and weeping with soaks is essential to quick resolution.

CASE STUDY

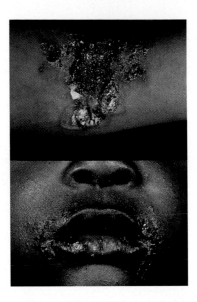

S: A 4-year-old black male presents to the clinic with his mother. She is worried about numerous ugly erosive sores around his nose and lips that have been spreading over the last 3 days. She has also noticed a similar rash on his right forearm. She says that about 5 days ago she found the patient playing "daddy" and using her husband's razor to shave. He had a few small cuts and abrasions on his face, which she washed with plain water and otherwise did not treat. No other complaints at this time.

O: *General*—Well nourished well fed, but poorly groomed child.
Skin—Multiple 1mm to 5mm diameter red, well-demarcated "satellite" plaques surround 2–4 cm well demarcated red, erosions at margins of lips and right anti-arbital fossa. There is a mild amount of yellowish crusting. A few tiny vesicles with clear contents are present as well.

A: Impetigo

P: Cool soaks with Hibclens at least twice each day; gently remove all crusts
   ▾ Bactroban ointment to area twice each day
   ▾ Clean his fingernails. Bathe him.
   ▾ Patient education on appropriate wound care and importance of good hygiene.
   ▾ Follow-up if no improvement in 5–7 days

PATIENT EDUCATION HANDOUT

PYODERMA

Keep all wounds—even small scratches—clean and dry.

Apply antibacterial ointment to wounds at least twice each day.
Avoid picking / scratching at any skin lesion.

If redness, swelling spreads despite antibiotics – SEE YOUR DOCTOR *IMMEDIATELY*.

Hot tubs often cause bacterial infection of the hair follicles.

If told to use soaks, apply cool water compress to lesions at least twice each day—better if every 3–4 hours.

Take all medication as directed until finished.

Keep your follow-up appointments if scheduled.

▶ Seborrheic Dermatitis

BACKGROUND

Seborrheic dermatitis is a chronic skin disease characterized by redness, pruritus, and scaling. The disease may present at infancy (known commonly as cradle cap) or puberty, but most patients with seborrheic dermatitis present at age 20 or older. Episodes of the disorder wax and wan throughout a patients lifetime. It is seen more commonly in males than in females.

The exact etiology of seborrheic dermatitis is not known. Moist conditions in hair-bearing skin due to sweating and poor grooming may play some role in its development. Infrequent cleaning of hairy of intertrigonal areas, the summer season, warm/humid climates, a high fat diet, alcohol ingestion, and severe fatigue are all known to exacerbate seborrheic dermatitis. Diseases that lead to facial flushing, such as acne rosacea, will worsen seborrheic dermatitis. Also, this skin disorder can appear or flare in association with diseases of the central nervous system. Degenerative CNS diseases, strokes, and brain trauma may directly induce seborrheic dermatitis.

IN THE CLINIC

Seborrheic dermatitis may be of two types: **sicca** or **oleosa**. The **sicca** type is a dry, white, flaky eczema-like process. It is often seen in persons with dry skin and atopic dermatitis. Individual lesions present as macules or papules with poor demarcation and overlying fine white scale. The **oleosa** form is a much more inflammatory process. It is seen in persons with oily skin types who may demonstrate severe acne or hidradenitis. Most scalp seborrhea is of the oleosa type. These lesions are also poorly defines macules or papules, but their color is usually yellowish-red with an overlying oily appearance. Scale is larger and usually yellowish in color. Sticky crusts, overt weeping, and fissures are often encountered.

The lesions of seborrheic dermatitis may occur on any areas of hair-bearing skin and often extend into adjacent non-hairy areas. They are most often encountered on the scalp, eyebrows, axilla, beard, behind the ears, forehead, groin, anogenital area, and submammary areas. The lesions are almost always pruritic in nature. Fortunately, the extent of the pruritus is very limited and secondary excoriation is rarely seen. Infants present with "cradle cap"—lesions of the sicca variety that occur on the infant's scalp. Often the entire scalp is involved, and the changes resemble a dry, white, flaking "cap." In this manifestation, the lesions occur in the first 3 months of life and most children have full resolution by 18 months of age. This infant form does not predispose a patient to develop seborrhea as an adult.

Most clinically diagnosed external otitis media is actually a complication of seborrheic dermatitis. Thus, it is of utmost importance that patients diagnosed with the external variety of otitis media be dissuaded from any behavior that might further aggravate the skin's trauma. This would include picking, digging, or the use of neomycin based ear drops. Also, seborrhea is very commonly seen in patients with AIDS. If a patient presents with severe and uncontrollable seborrheic dermatitis on the face, a diagnosis of AIDS should be considered.

DIAGNOSIS AND TREATMENT

The differential diagnosis of seborrheic dermatitis commonly includes psoriasis, dermatophytosis, and candidiasis. A KOH exam is often helpful in the clinical setting to quickly rule out a fungal origin. Also, lesions that simulate sebderm are seen in various nutritional deficiencies including both niacin and zinc deficiencies. As noted earlier, rosacea is often seen in the presence of the oleosa form of seborrheic dermatitis.

The first goal in treating seborrheic dermatitis is the removal of the overlying scale. This result is best achieved with persistent and frequent cleansing. The below cleansers should initially be applied every day and may be changed to every other day as improvement occurs. Cleansers include 1% to 5% salicylic acid lotion (choice for infants and children), Dermasmooth FS oil, and Baker's P & S liquid. Effective shampoos contain 5% selenium sulfide, tar, elemental sulfur, or ketoconazole. If involvement is extensive and severe, clobetasol propionate scalp solution may be used for short periods only.

Topical mid-potency steroids are often used in facial eruptions if the disease is more extensive, or if the above cleansers are not fully effective. These should be applied twice a day initially and when the disease is under better control may be switched to once a day or substituted with cleansers as above. If there exists any concomitant acne, rosacea, or pyoderma, these must be treated as well.

MANAGEMENT

To Manage

▼ Keep almost all cases

▼ Patient education of realistic results. Lesions will remit and exacerbate.

▼ First: **REMOVE THE SCALE**

▼ Cleanse frequently and persistently.

▼ Treat every day initially. May change to twice a day once lesions improve.

▼ Options include

1% to 5% Salicylic acid lotion (choice for infants)

Dermasmooth FS oil (esp. good if cornification)

Baker's P&S liquid

Selsun blue shampoo (in mild cases only)

5% Selenium sulfide shampoo

Tar shampoo

Elemental sulfur

Ketoconazole shampoo

▼ Facial involvement and second line after above-topical mid-potency steroids applied twice a day initially then decreased to once a day as improvement occurs.

▼ Treat all underlying disease, including acne, rosacea, or vasomotor disruptions.

Send

▼ Cases unresponsive to above

▼ Cases requiring biopsy

▼ Ulcerative or nodular cases

PROGNOSIS

The disease course is chronic with periods of exacerbation and remission. Treatment for each episode is quite effective, but patients must be warned that the lesions will more than likely reoccur. Infants with cradle cap do grow out of the disease and are not predisposed to adult forms.

PEARLS AND PITFALLS

▼ Patient education is important.

▼ Topical cleansers are best if left on 5–10 minutes a treatment.

▼ Treat any underlying skin disease—pyodermas, acne, rosacea, or vasomotor disease.

CASE STUDY

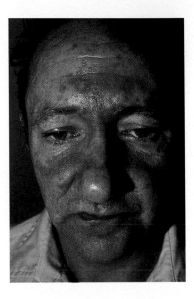

S: A 65-year-old male presents with a 4-month history of an itchy papulosquamous rash around his nose, chin and cheeks. He believed it to
be dry skin and has been applying over the counter facial lotion without any improvement. In fact, he feels that the rash has been worsening over the past few weeks. He otherwise has no complaints.

O: Skin—multiple erythematous papules and macules around his nasal
folds, cheeks, chin and forehead. These areas are well circumscribed
and have mid overlying yellowish scale. One lesion demonstrates a
small 3-mm fissure and there is evidence of weeping. The surrounding facial skin is slightly shiny in appearance. The nose itself is red as
well with multiple small pustules present. No excoriation is seen.

A: 1. Seborrheic Dermatitis
  2. Acne Rosacea

P: 1. Selenium sulfide 5%—apply two times a day for 2 weeks. If improvement, lesions may reduce to once a day after 2 weeks. If no
  improvement after 2 weeks, the patient should return to clinic. At
  this point, a 2-week trial of mid potency steroids twice a day. If still
  no improvement, consider dermatology referral.
  2. Topical cleocin or erythromycin twice a day with cleansing. See
  appropriate chapter.

PATIENT EDUCATION HANDOUT
SEBORRHEIC DERMATITIS

The skin disease you have has been diagnosed with is called *Seborrheic Dermatitis*.

This rash is treatable—but it may return at a later time. Things that cause it to return are the following:

Sweaty/wet skin
Stress (mental/physical)
Hot/humid climate
High fat diet
Alcohol
Not cleaning hairy skin/scalp often enough
Fatigue

Your child has a special type of this disease called "cradle cap" and will grow out of it without an increased chance of getting the same skin disease when older.

We have prescribed _____ to use on the skin.

Instructions on how to use this treatment are as follows:

_____

_____

_____

If the rash does not improve in 2 weeks or if it gets worse, call the office.

Call if any questions or concerns.

▶ URTICARIA AND ANGIOEDEMA

BACKGROUND

Urticaria and angioedema are characterized by various sized areas of skin edema. The swelling is limited to the dermis in urticaria while angioedema involves such changes in the subcutaneous tissues as well. Angioedema may or may not have associated urticarial lesions. These diseases are recurrent and can be acute and last minutes to days. But, they can also be chronic and last months to years. Most people experience urticara sometime in life.

Urticaria and angioedema can be either an immunologic or non-immunolgic phenomena. If immunologic, the etiology is usually IgE or complement mediated. Remember the IgE-mediated process is a type I hypersentivity reaction. An IgE antibody is formed to an inciting agent during initial exposure. This specific antibody is then attached to the membrane of mast cells. Thus, when reexposed to the specific agent, its antigen will bind two of these site-specific antibodies on the mast cell membrane. The antigen-antibody complex formation on the mast cell leads to its degranulation. The degranulation of mast cells via this process releases histamines causing the clinically observed changes of urticaria and angioedema. Examples of inciting antigens commonly include foods (fish, nuts, eggs, etc) and drugs (PCN, blood products). These individuals may have a history of atopy and often a serum IgE level will be elevated.

Most types of the physical urticarias are known to be pathophysiologically IgE mediated. The physical urticarias include cholinergic urticaria, cold urticaria, pressure urticaria and solar urticaria. Physical urticaria erupt repeatedly in the same locations on the skin, and often seasonally.

Cholinergic urticaria involves acetocholine in the IgE-mediated process but the details are still unknown. This subtype of physical urticaria occurs when exercise to the stage of sweating or hot baths provoke typical 3–5mm urticarial skin changes. Cold urticaria is common in children and occurs when the skin is exposed to cold stimuli. Placing a piece of ice on an individual suspected of having this form of the skin disease should produce the typical lesions within minutes. Solar urticaria occurs when a person develops urticarial lesions after exposure to certain wavelengths of ultraviolet light. Pressure urticaria/angioedema is a type of physical urticaria that involves edema more prominently than urticarial skin changes.

In this subtype, the presence of pressure leads to swelling and erythema of the areas of skin directly exposed to the traumatic force. Examples are dermatographism, or edema of the hand after catching a ball, or delayed urticaria of the feet in runners.

Complement-mediated etiologies involve a different immunologic phenomena. In this process, the antigen-antibody complex directly activities complement. This "turning on" of complement eventually leads to the release of various anaphylaxis agents. These agents then proceed to cause mast cell degranulation and the release of inflammatory mediators. Examples of this type of immunologic etiology include hereditary angioedema (autosomal dominant) and serum sickness.

Non-immunologic mechanisms that produce urticaria and angioedema include direct stimulation of mast cells via pharmacologic mechanisms (radio contrast media NSAIDS, ACE inhibitors, benzoates and the azoclyse tartrazile) and the induction of the lipoxygenase pathway of anaccidenic acid. These non-immunologic mechanisms are associated with the release of the same inflammatory mediators as are the IgE and complement related immunologic phenomena described above. There also exists a clan of urticaria/angioedema which is idiopathic. Unfortunately, these are the forms of this skin disease that are usually chronic in nature.

IN THE CLINIC

Urticaria presents as pale to erythematous papules, plaques or wheals (up to 8cm diameter). The lesions are extremely well demarcated from surrounding unaffected skin. The actual shape of each lesion can vary from round, to oval to serpiginous. Urticaria may be localized to one specific region of the body or may be generalized. Urticaria are both pruritic and transient. A specific lesion will last no more than 24 hours and usually shows some migration within 2–4 hours. But other lesions may occur on other skin areas during an outbreak. Specific wheals that last >12 hours are indicative of a disease other than urticaria. Take a thorough history to rule out repeated attacks due to repeated exposure to drugs or physical agents. The remaining non-transient "urticaria-like" lesions are commonly indicative of an underlying illness such as necrotizing vasculitis, chronic lower bowel disease, histoplasma, tuberculosis, neoplasm, hyperthyroidism, regional enteritis, and giardiasis. As noted previously, urticarial outbreaks that persist 6 weeks or less are acute. Chronic urticaria is seen as similar recurrent attacks that continue over more than 6 weeks.

Angioedema may be present with urticaria or may occur without any of these more superficial lesions. As mentioned previously, this disease involves non-pitting edema of the deeper layers of the skin and of subcutaneous tissues. The huge hive-like swellings have poor margination and no color change of the overlying epidermis. The face genitalia and extremities are commonly affected.

A very rare autosomally dominant inherited disorder known as hereditary angioedema occurs in the absence of any urticaria. This autosomally dominant disease is typified by painful angioedema of the face, bowel, larynx, and extremities. The edema may last up to 2–4 days. Extensive areas are usually involved and this nonallergic phenomena may be fatal.

DIAGNOSIS AND TREATMENT

The diagnosis of urticaria and angioedema is usually based solely on patient history and clinical presentation. If the history is thorough, the etiology of the skin reaction is usually readily apparent. Keep in mind while taking a history that many viral syndromes can include skin changes that appear urticarial. Thus, be sure to rule out a febrile exanthem as the true etiology. Other common diseases included in the differential diagnosis of urticaria include erythema multiforme, early herpes simplex, early herpes zoster, and insect bite reactions.

If urticaria are persistent, and repetitive exposure to an allergin is ruled out, one must search for a possible underlying illness. Try to decide if the patient is ill, in terms of fever, weight loss, malaise or a notable review of systems. In cases of illness with chronic urticaria CBC, sedimentation rate, liver function test, $TSHT_4$ urinalysis, stool for ova and parasites, and culture of any possible abscess or infection locus are useful. A carefully selected skin biopsy of a lesion lasting > 24 hours may reveal vasculitis. Often complement levels and ANA testing prove fruitful in cases of angioedema.

As previously mentioned, most urticaria are acute and no specific therapy is indicated. Treatment of these patients includes measures to reduce pruritus as well as patient education to avoid any inciting allergens. Anti-pruritic measures include cool water or Burow's solution soaks as well as oral antihistamines (hydroxizine, diphenhydramine, terfenadine, astemizole, etc). Topical mid-potency corticosteroids up to three times daily can be helpful, but if wide areas of skin are involved, their application is not always practical.

If the urticaria is a physical (cholinergic) type both topical steroids and antihistamines may also be helpful. A few individuals recommend desensitization therapy. This method of treatment involves desensitization of the individual to the physical stimulus via exposure to gradually increasing amounts of said stimulus.

Chronic severe urticaria are also treated with high dose antihistamines. Again, look for evidence of an underlying physical illness.

Severe urticaria and angioedema may require systemic corticosteroid treatment. Before initiating such therapy be certain to rule out any possible infection as the etiology. Use a tapered regimen over 10 days to 2 weeks. Phase in adequate antihistamine therapy.

Hereditary angioedema is treated acutely with subcutaneous epinephrine and fresh frozen plasma. Prophylaxis can be accomplished via oral Danazol at doses of 200 mg three times daily with a taper of 30% every 2 months. Without treatment, these episodes episodically increase in severity until they may cultimate in death.

MANAGEMENT

To Manage

▼ Keep all acute urticaria/angioedema without anaphylaxis.

▼ Those chronic urticaries with known allergens

▼ Chronic urticarias requiring initial lab investigation.

To Treat

▼ Improve pruritus

1. Cool water soaks 2 to 3 times a day

2. Oral antihistamines (hydroxyzine, or nonsedating varieties) as needed.

▼ Topical mid-potency steroid twice-a-day to affected areas, especially for urticaria in atopics.

▼ If severe or facial/genital involvement:

1. Oral steroids taper over 10–14 days.

Send

Any suspected anaphylaxis to emergency room immediately.

Chronic urticarias that are fixed or with exceptional lab work up for collaborative discussion/biopsy.

Hereditary angioedema patients.

PROGNOSIS

The vast majority of all urticaria and angioedema will resolve spontaneously without any therapy. If an episode is severe, therapy is often indicated and the prognosis remains excellent. Hereditary angioedema has a natural course of progressively worsening without the initiation of prophylactic therapy. It will eventually end in a severe anaphylaxic episode and death if medical intervention is not sought. All anaphylaxis may be fatal if therapy is not initiated. But, once therapy is started, the majority of these reactions have an excellent prognosis.

PEARLS AND PITFALLS

- ▼ Use systemic corticosteroids only in those patients with severe symptoms or involvement of the face and/or genitalia.
- ▼ Any patient with possible anaphylaxis should seek emergency medical care immediately.
- ▼ Take a thorough history to determine the probable inciting allergen and advise patient to avoid this agent. Have a protocol ready to implement in the ER.
- ▼ If a patient has urticarial-like lesions that are fixed (ie. Non-migratory) the probable etiology is vasculitis and a biopsy should be performed promptly.
- ▼ Chronic reoccurring or persistent lesions without obvious source of allergin require lab work up and possible biopsy.
- ▼ Look for tiny purpura in the center of urticarial bug bites.

CASE STUDY

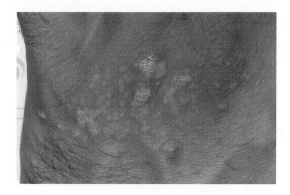

S: A patient arrives in your outpatient clinic with a 1 day history of an "itchy-rash." He is a natural bodybuilder and has a competition in 2 days and is worried he will not get rid of the rash before then. He knows he cannot win the event if his skin is "red and blotchy." He denies any such rash in the past and states he is not short of breath, no chest pain or dysphagia. He admits to no new foods or activities. He does use tanning salons two times a week in his attempt to "stay healthy looking" for his competition.He admits to such artificial tanning for 2 3 years and has not used any new facilities or topical tanning products. He does admit to taking two "pain pills" the previous day for his sore muscles. He bummed these off of a friend which he has done once in the past as well. He cannot remember the name of the medication but calls his lifting buddy who tells him it was a nonsteroidal anti-inflammatory drug. He has no further useful history. He denies use of anabolic steroids.

O: General: Patient is a young, well-developed white male in no respiratory distress.

Skin: Diffuse 1–5 cm diameter erythematous plaques with central white pallor. These are widely distributed over the face, trunk, arms, and legs. The skin also shows urticaria in folds not exposed to UV and some mild excoriation—some over areas where none of these lesions appear. No scale or other secondary changes. No evidence of acne-like pustules/papules.

H25NT: Lips and perioral area are slightly edematous but not tender to palpation. Rest is wir. No changes of mucous membranes are seen.

Lump: CTA B

CV: $S_1 + S_2$ without mummer S_3-RRR. Peripheral pulses full and equal bilaterally.

Abd: benign

A: Urticaria and perioral/lip angioedema.

Most likely secondary to NSAID ingestion

P: 1. Avoid NSAID—list examples for the patient.
2. Cool water soaks 3 times a day or until itching resolves.
3. Oral antihistamine every 8 hours as needed for pruritus.
4. Patient advised about the actually "unhealthy" glow he received from use of tanning salons.
5. If any change in ability to breath/swallow or other new symptoms, phone or seek medical attention immediately.

PATIENT EDUCATION HANDOUT
URTICARIA AND ANGIOEDEMA

Your doctor has diagnosed your rash as "hives" or a skin reaction that is usually due to an allergy.

This allergy may be due to food, medicine, temperatures, viruses, and many other causes. Your physician believes your rash may be due to _____.

Avoid this substance at all times.

If your reaction is severe and you become short of breath or have problems swallowing, seek medical attention immediately.

If you have had reactions where you become short of breath or have problems swallowing you may have these again if exposed to the same allergen. Ask your doctor about "epinephrine" and how to get a kit for your home in case of an emergency.

Most of these rashes without any breathing/swallowing problems get better on their own.

If your rash itches:

- ▼ Cool wash cloths to rash or cool tap water baths as needed.
- ▼ Keep your skin "well lotioned" with a hypoallergenic cream. Your doctor suggests _____.
- ▼ Ask your doctor about medicine to take by mouth that will improve the itching.
- ▼ If your rash returns again or does not get better in 1 month, let your doctor know. He/she may want to look further at other possible reasons this is happening.

▶ WARTS: VERRUCA VULGARIS AND CONDYLOMA

BACKGROUND

All warts are simply benign hyperplasia of the epithelium. The global term "warts" encompasses the following entities—flat warts (verruca plana), common warts (verruca vulgaris), periungual warts, plantar warts (verruca plantaris), and genital, oral and anal warts (condyloma acuminata). The skin changes seen with warts are caused by the papova group of human wart virus called human papilloma virus. Each of the above types of warts are due to a different papovavirus. Every wart sheds virus locally on the skin and satellite lesions can form and initiate spread of the skin disease. Biting on a wart may spread them to lips or into the mouth.

Warts are most commonly seen in children and young adults (5–25 years) although they may appear in almost any age group. Spread between individuals can and frequently does occur. This transmission can be sexual (as in condyloma acuminata), nonsexual skin-to-skin, or via fomites. All warts are more common and widespread in an immunocompromised patient. Further description of each of the clinical manifestations of the papovaviruses follows in the next section.

IN THE CLINIC

Almost all warts begin as tiny pale papules without inflammation. These eventually enlarge to 5–10mm in diameter while maintaining their basic lichen morphology. Flat warts (verruca plana) are usually seen in young children but can also be demonstrated in adults (mostly females). They present as 1–5-mm papules that are often seen in distinct clusters. They are minimally raised with flat tops and are usually flesh colored or light brown. Flat warts appear most commonly on the dorsum of the hands and shaved areas such as the face in men and the legs in women. Often, the lesions can appear in a linear configuration due to scratching and autoinoculation. These lesions have a tendency to appear around follicles.

Common warts (verruca vulgaris) are also common in young children, but are seen more often in females than males. These well-demarcated papules are round to square in shape, flesh colored, and usually 1 to 10 mm in diameter. Close inspection of these lesions will demonstrate characteristics of tiny black dots which represent thrombosed capillary loops. These warts will develop on "pressure-free," dry skin surfaces and have a predilection for sites of trauma such as the finger joints, hands, under fingernails and on the knees. Although these are the most usual places one will find common warts, they may appear anywhere on the body. The warts may be seen as individual lesions but they are often grouped in clusters. Common warts demonstrate the same autoinoculation properties as flat warts and these may be spread in scratches.

Periungual warts are a variety of common warts and display the clinical characteristics previously described. But, these warts are characterized by their location. They grow into the skin folds around the nail bed and are most commonly seen in those patients who bite their nails. These warts may grow to a size where they erode underlying bone and can lead to a pathologic fracture.

Genital warts (condyloma acuminata) are those HPV induced skin changes that occur on wet epithelial surfaces such as on the genital anal and oral mucosa. They are usually found in sexually active young adults. These lesions are the most contagious of all warts and various strains are oncogenic in nature. The typical lesions in mouth and throat are white papules or plaques. The genital and anal areas demonstrate lesions that are fleshy-colored and may range from 1 mm in diameter to large cauliflower or sea sponge like masses. Genital warts can be present but not visualized to the naked eye. These lesions will become apparent with acetowhitening. Condyloma acuminata can appear any where on the genital-rectal area, periurthera, urethral meatus, bladder, perianal skin, anal canal, lips, mouth, or throat. The preponderance of genital warts has increased dramatically in the last 10 years and more than 90% of partners of an infected female will acquire the virus.

Planter warts (verruca plantaris) can be seen at any age and in either sex, but are most common in 5 to 25-year-old females. At the outset of eruption, these lesions are small, flesh-colored papules with well-demarcated margins. They occur on the plantar surface of the feet, especially over the metatarsal heads, heel, and toes. These areas are subjected to significant pressure and secondary trauma. The constant pressure of walking can lead to overlying callus formation and secondary indentation of the wart itself. Thus what often appears clinically to be a callus should be pared down to visualize the black dots characteristic of a plantar wart. These warts, like the common variety discussed earlier, can contain thrombosed capillary loops that are seen as these black dots and are not found in other hyperkeratotic lesions. All plantar warts are tender to palpation; some may be almost disabling in nature.

DIAGNOSIS AND TREATMENT

Almost all warts are easily diagnosed via just their clinical presentation. Genital warts can be subclinical and may need acetowhitening to visualize. This process involves applying gauze soaked with a 5% acetic acid solution to the area in question of 5 minutes. A hand lens or colposcope is then employed to demonstrate the papules. Plantar and common warts should demonstrate the black dots of thrombosed capillary loops (remember to pare down any overlying callus). Treatment of warts depends on where they clinically present as outlined:

a. *Flat warts*—these usually spontaneously clear in a short time period. If the patient is concerned or if they present a cosmetic issue, one may use Retinoic Acid 0.5% once daily for 2 to 4 weeks. Cryotherapy or electrosurgery are options but definitely overkill.

b. *Common warts*—these lesions can be treated with a 40% salicylic acid solution in plaster or colloidin form. This mixture should be applied daily for up to 6 weeks. Cryotherapy for 10 to 30 seconds every 2 weeks until clearing is also an acceptable treatment. These lesions can also be removed via laser surgery.

c. *Genital/Perianal warts*—these skin changes are best treated with cryotherapy for 10 to 30 seconds. Again, multiple treatments at 2 to 3 week intervals may be necessary. Podophyllin may be employed if liquid nitrogen is unavailable. This solution is potentially toxic so the physician should treat only small areas (<10 c) at a time and it should never be used in pregnant patients. An alternative is 0.5% Podophilex for patient self-treatment of lesions. Directions should be given to apply the liquid to the warts twice a day for 3 days then no treatment for 4 days then twice a day for 3 days, etc . . . . for a total of 4 weeks. A final option is electrocautery or laser surgery.

d. *Anal warts*—cryosurgery for 10 to 30 seconds. Retreat every 2 to 3 weeks until resolved. Electrosurgery or laser surgery are options if cryotherapy fails.

e. *Oral warts*—same as for anal warts as outlined.
f. *Paronychial warts*—these lesions respond poorly to the standard treatment of other common warts. The preferred method of treatment is via DNCB. This therapy involves injecting intralesional interferon. It is effective in treating periwinkle warts.
g. *Plantar warts*—like flat warts these hyperkeratotic skin abnormalities show a high rate of spontaneous cure. Never treat a plantar wart that is asymptomatic. If symptoms are present, first pare off any overlying callus that has formed without actually excising the wart itself. Then apply the 40% salicylic acid collodion daily for up to 6 weeks or employ cryotherapy for 10 to 30 seconds every 2 to 3 weeks until cure. After treatment the key to quick resolution and prevention of reoccurrence is via decreasing pressure via padding, orthotics, or metatarsal bars. Laser and electrosurgery can be used as well, but are discouraged due to the possibility of creating a permanent, painful scar in an attempt to treat a lesion that if left alone will resolve spontaneously.

MANAGEMENT

To Manage

▼ Keep almost all cases

a) Flat warts—Patient education about spontaneous cure

Retin A 0.5% once a day for 2 to 4 weeks

Cryotherapy if necessary but usually overkill

b) Common warts—Keratolytics: 40% salicylic acid in plaster or collodion

Apply once a day for up to 6 weeks

Cryotherapy 10–30 seconds every 2 to 3 weeks until resolution

c) Genital warts—Podophyllin to small areas (<10 c) every 2 weeks

Podophylex 0.5% twice each day for 3 days then off for 4 days. Repeat for a total of 4 weeks.

Cryotherapy is proffered method—10 to 60 seconds every 2 to 3 weeks until resolved.

d) Oral warts—Cryotherapy 10 to 30 seconds every 2–3 weeks until resolved.

e) Anal warts—Cryotherapy 10 to 30 seconds every 2–3 weeks until resolved.

f) Planter warts—All will spontaneously cure.

First pare down any overlying callus.

Keratolytics: 40% salicylic acid in plaster or collodion.

Apply once a day for up to 6 weeks.

Cryotherapy 10 to 30 seconds every 2–3 weeks until resolved.

▼ Padding, metatarsal bars, and other methods to decrease pressure on the affected areas.

Send

▼ Periungual warts for DNCB treatment, laser surgery or electro-cautery

▼ Common or genital warts that are very large or do not respond to conservative treatment as outlined

▼ Immunosuppressed patients with multiple lesions

PROGNOSIS

Common and flat warts all have an excellent prognosis. Genital/anal/oral warts will reoccur in most patients even after appropriate treatment has been administered. This reoccurrence is due to the HPV lying in a dormant form on what appears to be normal skin next to the actual lesion.

PEARLS AND PITFALLS

▼ Never use Podophyllin of Podophilex in pregnant patients.

▼ Do not over treat plantar warts or common warts at the expense of producing a painful scar.

▼ Pare the callus off the top of a plantar wart, but be careful not to excise any of the wart itself.

▼ The HPV associated with genital warts has an increased risk of producing malignancy, so stress the importance of annual Pap tests to detect cervical dysplasia.

▼ Children delivered to mothers with apparent condyloma accuminta are at an increased risk of developing warts.

▼ An individual may demonstrate genital warts at a time well removed from when the HPV was transmitted. The virus can lay inert for a long period of time before producing the actual lesion. This notion is important in counseling your patient and their partner as to when this sexually transmitted disease was contracted.

CASE STUDY

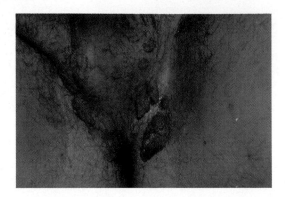

S: A 22-year-old female college student presents to the student health clinic with a 1-week history of non-painful but "bothersome" lesion on her genital region. She states she has been in a monogamous relationship for 6 months. She has never seen a lesion on her partner but admits to "not always looking." She does tell you that she has a part-time job as a dancer in a local mens club and is worried because other girls who work there have similar lesions. She asks if there is any way she could have "caught" whatever she has from shared towel or "the pole." She denies any anal intercourse but states she does engage in oral sex. She is otherwise without any complaints.

O: The left labia majora demonstrates a 5-mm, flesh-colored lesion that is well demarcated from the surrounding skin. The surface of the lesion is mildly filiform in appearance. There is no evidence of trauma or excoriation. A full examination of all anogenital and oral skin demonstrates no further skin changes.

A: Genital wart (condyloma acuminata)

P: Cryotherapy for 10–30 seconds every 2 to 3 weeks until resolved. If continues without improvement for over 6 weeks consider referral for laser or electrosurgery. Educate patient about the unlikelihood she contracted the disease from a fomite such as a shared towel or the "bar." Inform her that this disease does not mean her boyfriend has been unfaithful to her. Explain that the virus may have been in place on her own skin for many months or years before the lesions appeared. Also her partner may have the virus on this skin but not have any actual lesions. See another friend's similar condyloma, above.

S: A 32-year-old female hand model presents to your Beverly Hill Family Practice Clinic. She complains of multiple small lesions on her right hand which have been present for about 1 week. She is aghast at their appearance for she relies on her hand as an income source. She has no further complaints.

O: Skin on the dorsum of the right hand demonstrates 6 tightly clustered flesh-colored, flat-topped papules. Each papule is 3–4 mm in diameter. There exists no surrounding erythema, excoriation, or scale. Rest of the skin is without abnormality.

A: Flat warts

P: Although you explain to the patient that these warts will heal on their own in a few weeks to months, she insists on treatment due to her needing perfect hands in order to maintain her livelihood. Due to possible scarring with cryotherapy of electrosurgery you opt to treat with Retinoic acid 0.5% once a day for 2–4 weeks.

PATIENT EDUCATION HANDOUT
WARTS

Most warts on nongenital areas will resolve even without treatment.

If using a salicylic acid plaster, apply one time each day. It may take up to 6 weeks for a cure.

If using podophylex, apply once each day for 3 days then no treatment for 4 days then once a day for 3 days then no treatment for 4 days. Continue this repetition for a total of 4 weeks.

Keep all follow-up appointments with your physician as scheduled.

Treatment of warts can be painful but if you are experiencing a lot of severe pain you must inform your physician.

If you had a plantar wart treated today, keep area well padded each day until your physician sees you again. This padding is required if you want the wart to heal.

CHAPTER 6

OTHER COMMON DISORDERS

▶ ## ALOPECIA (HAIR LOSS)

BACKGROUND

Hair has no vital function, but of immeasurable psychological importance in both men and women. Alopecia is a common problem and is often quite distressing to the patient. A well-prepared collaborative plan by the primary care physician can serve to allay a patient's worry via early diagnosis with quick institution of a formal treatment plan. Remember though, these patients require extra time to reassure due to the cosmetic concern involved with hair loss.

Most hair is composed of elongated keratinized cells cemented together. Keratin itself is a group of insoluble protein helixes linked via a disulfide bond. Each keratinized hair shaft arises from a follicle. A single follicle will progress through 10 to 20 "hair cycles" in a lifetime. These natural cycles encompass a period of growth and activity (anagen phase) followed by a short transitional period (catagen phase) and finally, a period of rest (telogen phase). The duration of each phase depends on a number of factors including season, age, sex, and hormonal factors to name a few. These facts are important in an attempt to distinguish a normal pattern of hair loss from a pathologic form. Different types of alopecia will be discussed in more detail in the section that follows.

IN THE CLINIC

First, start with a detailed history—when did the alopecia begin? What areas began first? Does the scalp itch? This information lays an important base for diagnosis. Then move on to the physical examination. Look at the general picture—frontally (eye level) and down from above (the vertex) to determine an overall pattern. Draw pictures and record where appropriate. Decide how severe the overall loss is and whether it is patchy or diffuse. Are there any existing concomitant scalp disorders such as psoriasis or seborrheic dermatitis? Feel the hair's texture to determine if it has areas of thinning that we know often preceded frank alopecia. Now examine hair with a magnifying glass. Determine if the hairs are being broken off or if the loss is at the level of the cuticle. Broken hairs have no terminal bulb. If broken off, is the remaining hair shaft short or long? All of these details are important in forming the final diagnosis.

Now, *palpate* the scalp itself. Is the alopecia scarring in nature? Scarring alopecia is less common than its non-scarring counter part, more serious, and often requires a biopsy to determine the exact etiology. Scarring alopecia is permanent. The hair cannot regrow because the follicle has been destroyed. While palpating be certain to note any underlying lymph node involvement. A thorough physical exam as above is essential and should be focused on with attention to the history.

DIAGNOSIS AND TREATMENT

Many etiologies of alopecia exist, but in this text, we will focus on the 10 most common causes of alopecia. All of these are nonscarring entities and their clinical diagnoses and treatment will be outlined together to enable easier reading and quicker reference.

Therefore, there are two general types of hair loss—patchy and diffuse. Patchy loss can be scarring or non-scarring in form. Below the 12 most common etiologies of hair loss are discussed in greater detail.

Diffuse Loss
1. Male/female pattern baldness
2. Hypothyroidism
3. Drug effects
4. Postpartum telogen effluvium

5. Post-illness telogen effluvium
6. Underlying dermatitis of the scalp

Patchy Loss—Without Scar

7. Alopecia areata
8. Trichotillomania
9. Traction alopecia
10. Mild-moderate tinea capitis

Patchy Loss—with Scar

11. Severe tinea capitis
12. Bacterial infections of the scalp especially with acne component.

Tinea capitis is seen most often in children, but also can occur in adult patients. This form is characterized by raggedly demarcated patches of hair loss resembling "moth holes" in fabric. Individual hairs are usually broken off at the surface of the scalp leaving the area of complete or partial alopecia with a pattern of black dots at the scalp surface. These punctate marks are seen among crusts where the hair was originally present. Almost all scalp tinea is inflammatory and the hair loss is associated with varying degrees of scalp erythema and edema. One method to confirm the diagnosis of tinea is by KOH preparation (see appropriate section for details on how to perform this test). If in context with the clinical exam, hyphae/spores are present upon KOH exam, then the patient can be treated immediately. Because the treatment of tinea capitis is an oral antifungal drug with multiple possible side effects, it is vital that some definite evidence of fungal infection is in hand before treatment is begun. If the KOH is not diagnostic yet the clinical diagnosis continues to appear most reasonable, a fungal culture must be performed to ensure proper diagnosis before initiating oral antifungal therapy. Because fungal cultures are most cost-beneficial if done by gross morphology, it is necessary to arrange to have this performed by the dermatologist. Thus, these patients with a negative KOH but clinically probable tinea capitis should be referred to a dermatologist for confirmation and fungal culture. If the culture is positive, oral antifungal therapy should be started and the patient sent back to the primary care physician for continued therapy and follow-up.

Topical antifungals are never suitable for treating tinea capitis anymore due to many infective agents not fluorescing as hoped. Oral griseofulvin is very effective, and inexpensive. Proper treatment early usually results in full regrowth of hair. A high dose must be employed (750 mg–1g) each day in 3 divided dose (adults) and 7.5 mg/kg/day in three divided doses (children). *Never underdose.* Treatment is for a minimum of 8–12 weeks, but should be adjusted for each case. Remember to always give griseofulvin with food to avoid the side effect of nausea.

Alopecia areata—this very common type of hair loss results in sharply marginated patches of alopecia that are "velvety-soft" to touch. These patches are not inflamed and usually 2–3 cm in diameter. No scaling or infection is present. Each hair breaks off 2–3 mm above the scalps surface and the individual hair appears as "exclamation points" (Thick at top and thinner near the scalp). The remainder of the hair shows no thinning. Patients commonly present with one to three of these patches, but may have more. Rarely, total loss of hair results (alopecia totalis) but, loss in scalp only is most common. Eyebrows, lashes, beards, axilla, and pubic areas can be affected as well as the scalp and this is a dire prognostic finding. The exact etiology of this disease is not known. The general health of the patient is not affected, although the loss of hair can cause the patient great anxiety, and alopecia areata can lead to serious psychological problems.

Alopecia areata usually occurs in late childhood to early teen years and is more common in females than males. Twenty-five percent of patients have a family history of alopecia areata. The course of the disease is highly variable. Those patients that go into full remission usually have experienced about 6–12 months of progressively increasing hair loss, which then stabilizes for 6–12 months. After this time new hairs start to regrow (initially white in color) and hair returns to previous state by 1¹⁄₂ to 2 years. The time span is a burden to patients; they need plenty of reassurance and encouragement. Those patients who achieve complete remission still usually have a small number of tiny patches of original hair loss. The smaller and fewer the original patches the better the prognosis for full spontaneous remission.

Treatment options include high dose topical steroids twice a day (with optional nighttime shower cap occlusion) or intralesional steroids. Unfortunately, no treatment has been shown to be demonstrably better than placebo in regard to the final outcome. Thus, patient education and reassurance are the primary goals in treatment.

Trichotillomania—this form of hair loss also presents in a patchy distribution in most cases. But in this disease the patches may be huge. The hairs typically are broken within 1 cm from the scalp. This disease can occur in children or adults. Since there exists no underlying scalp disease, hairs continue to grow. The etiology is purely psychological-anxiety which leads to habitual pulling, chronic twisting, or frequent rubbing of a localized patch of hair. Trichotillomania may be a component of obsessive-compulsive personality disorder. Treatment consists of counseling and possible psycho-pharmacotherapy, but the first goal in primary care is to rule-out other possible etiologies for the hair loss.

Male/female pattern baldness—a familial "curse" of hair loss at an early age, which occurs in a characteristically diffuse pattern. The degree of hair loss and time in life at which it presents are both inherited. Males usually present with vertex loss and/or bitemporal loss from age 18 and up. Females demonstrate a vertex/generalized pattern which begins usually at age 50 and older but may be seen in the thirties. Hair loss is not constant over time—rather it occurs sporadically with intermittent periods of no noticeable hair loss. Treatment may include minoxidil (Rogaine) which can lead to a small amount of regrowth. Hair transplants may be desirable in a few cases, but are very expensive.

Excessive traction of the hair can lead to patchy, non-scarring alopecia. This form of hair loss is seen frequently in black patients or others who have tightly braided hairdos. Hard brushing, styling rollers and other fashion tricks often cause hair loss. Tension on the hair follicle can cause subsequent damage and prolonged loss of hair. This form of alopecia is best treated via prevention. Hair should not be braided on extremely tight styles and, if braided, should not remain so for long time periods. Proper patient education is the key and prevention is the cure.

Severe dermatitis of the scalp can cause alopecia as well. Allergic eczema and irritant dermatitis can cause hair loss. Seborrheic dermatitis is a common eczema-like disease. Seborrheic inflammation causes a diffuse hair loss. Also, although psoriasis does not in itself cause hair loss, it can lead to secondary alopecia. *(See the sections that outline these specific diseases for therapy guidelines.)*

Post partum telogen effluvium—Unlike most other mammals, humans don't have cyclic heavy shedding, but constantly rotate individual hairs through a growth cycle (anagen) and a resting period (telogen) in which the hair is discarded. The resting period is 3–4 months long, while anagen is 2 to 20 years depending on age, health, inheritance, and other causes. During pregnancy, for instance, all hairs push into anagen phase. The hair is uncommonly thick. But when pregnancy ends, the "telogen debt" becomes due and a considerable amount of hair can be lost. Some women will notice alarming thinning. A baby goes through the same cycle of hair growth and loss. Recovery may take a full year, possibly 2 years to recover full "thickness" or texture. Other causes of sudden diffuse hair loss (hypothyroidism, malnutrition, fever, drug effects, trichotillomania, etc) should always be considered and ruled out. Treatment is solely via patient education and reassurance. Obviously, suppression of adrenals with Decadron is counterindicated. Almost all of these patients eventually recover entirely. The problem improves with management of the anxiety the patient feels due to the hair loss.

Post illness telogen effluvium—anyone severely burdened by illness will also convert hair from anagen phase to telogen phase. Thus, 3–4 months from the incident, hair will be shed, only to begin to grow again after a pause of an additional 2–6 months. Remember thickness and "texture" may not be regained for an additional 2 years. Shedding may be quite severe and hair thickness may be reduced by almost one-half, but usually less thinning is involved. Prolonged anesthesia, influenza, infectious mononucleosis, and hepatitis are good examples of a medical crisis sufficient to cause a telogen hair loss. Also, severe accidents can cause telogen hair loss. Always examine the scalp carefully to determine that no other new primary lesions of the skin have appeared. These patients require no treatment, but as in the postpartum lots of reassurance is always indicated.

Drug effects—a variety of therapeutic agents can cause alopecia as a side effect. This form of alopecia is almost exclusively diffuse in nature with no underlying scalp changes. The most common drugs implicated are oncological agents. Other drugs, include Accutane, methotrexate, vitamin A, prednisone, heparin, thallium, Levodopa, to name a few. The most common therapeutic cause of diffuse alopecia is the birth control pill, but the loss occurs when the patient *stops* the medication. This alopecia usually occurs approximately 3 months after the oral contraceptives are discontinued and patients should be forewarned. Treatment includes discontinuing the medication and reassurance. Full regrowth will occur.

Hypothyroidism—this cause of alopecia also demonstrates a diffuse pattern of hair loss. It is more common in females with hypothyroidism than males with the same hormone deficiency. The mechanism behind the loss of hair is not known. Unfortunately, it may not be *directly* related to the lack of hormone, and so we see a lack of improvement of alopecia with thyroid hormonal replacement. Patients with hair loss invariably show multiple signs of a deficient thyroid gland such as decreased vigor, memory flaws, cold intolerance, sleepiness, weight gain and other problems. No specific treatment has yet proven effective.

If it is obvious to the diagnostic eye that underlying skin lesions accompany the alopecia, then hypothyroidism, alopecia areata, male/female pattern baldness, trichotillomania, and traction are probably not the correct diagnosis. Tinea, psoriasis, and seborrheic dermatitis are much more likely in patients with accompanying scalp lesions. Rarely, discoid lupus may be involved. If the diagnosis is in question, a biopsy may prove helpful. Biopsies are most cost effective when done by or in phone consultation with a dermatology. Also, lymphoma and scalp metastasis can cause alopecia, but these are accompanied by palpable plaques, lumps, and masses.

MANAGEMENT

To Manage

Keep almost all.

▼ Tinea Capitis

Adults—oral griseofulvin—330 mg of ultramicrosize form in 3 divided doses for 8–12 weeks.

Children—7.5 mg/kg/day in 3 divided doses for 8–12 weeks.

▼ Dermatitis of Scalp—treat underlying disease.

(psoriasis/seb dermatitis/ etc) as per appropriate text chapter.

▼ Alopecia Areata

High dose topical steroids BID for 6–12 weeks.

Possible addition of shower cap occlusion.

Intralesional steroids if above fails.

Patient education/reassurance.

▼ Trichotillomania

Rule out other possible etiologies

Counseling

Psychopharmacotherapy

▼ Hypothyroidism
  Correct thyroid deficiency
  Hair loss possible permanent—ie patient education/reassurance.
▼ Male/female pattern baldness
  Minoxidil
  Hair transplants
  Realistic expectation
▼ Traction
  Loosen braids/ponytails
  Prevention via patient education

Send

▼ If difficult diagnosis, for second opinion or biopsy.
▼ Clinically suspect T. capitis with negative KOH for fungal culture before initiating oral griseofulvin.
▼ Scarring forms
▼ Palpable bumps/lumps on scalp—for biopsy to rule out cancer metastasis or furuncles.
▼ Unremitting pyodermas
▼ Loss of eyelashes

PROGNOSIS

The prognosis of alopecia depends entirely on its etiology. Please refer to the above text on each specific form of hair loss. Remember the importance of patient education with hair loss because this problem can be quite psychologically stressful.

PEARLS AND PITFALLS

▼ Patient education is a key element.
▼ Dandruff does not cause hair loss.
▼ Hair directly reflects the overall health of the patient.
▼ Hair care is discussed in the cosmetics chapter.
▼ Be realistic with the patient—let them know the treatment options and be honest if no treatment is beneficial.

CASE 6.1

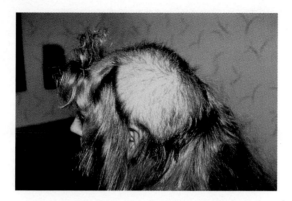

S: A healthy 35-year-old female presents with a 12 x 10 cm diameter area of hair loss on occipital scalp. She has no complaints of itching, previous hair loss, familial hair loss, and is on no medication. She is employed as a surgical scrub nurse and states her job is stressful. She is recently divorced and has just found out her 15-year-old daughter is pregnant and planning to drop out of school to marry the baby's father—a 25-year-old lead base guitarist for a local grunge band—"The Rocket Scientists."

O: General—an anxious female who cannot stop moving and appears to have pressured speech. She sleeps poorly and is always tired. Skin—scalp demonstrates a poorly demarcated 5 cm diameter patch of hair loss. Hair is broken off irregularly with 1/2–1 cm fragments remaining. The underlying skin is normal and without erythema on scale. Her nails demonstrate irregular edges and appear to have been bitten. Rest of exam—WNL

A: Trichotillomania

P: Check a TSH on this patient to rule out thyroid disorder. Give the patient attention and treat like a physiological hair loss. Have patient return in 2 weeks for results of lab test. Talk further about her stressful life and explore further her anxious state. Once patient has admitted to anxiety, explain hair loss can be a manifestation of anxiety and discuss further pharmacotherapy and counseling. It is often not advisable to accuse patient of "pulling out" hair. They will become defensive and you will alienate the individual. Treat as a real disease with plenty of reassurance. This goal often takes multiple visits and a significant amount of time.

CASE 6.2

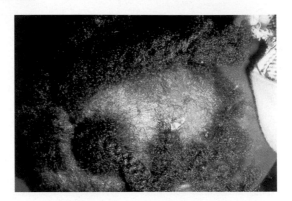

S: A 5-year-old black female presents with her mother. She has a 2-cm diameter patch of hair loss on her right temporal region. Her mother states she is constantly itching this area and the loss has occurred over the past 2 weeks.

O: Her hair is tightly braided. There is a well-circumscribed area of hair loss 2 cm in diameter on the right temporal region. There are no broken hairs evident. The underlying scalp is erythematous, mildly edematous, crusted and profusely scaling.

You perform a KOH which is negative.

A: Probable tinea capitis.

P: This patient requires confirmation of Tinea before starting treatment. Thus, send the patient to the dermatologist for fungal culture.

Fungal culture is positive.

Dermatologist starts patient on 7.5 mg/kg/day of oral ultramicrosize griseofulvin in 3 divided doses and sends patient back to you.

You monitor her progress every 4 weeks and keep her on the medication for 8–12 weeks total. Repeat the culture at 8 weeks and send bottle to your dermatologist.

PATIENT EDUCATION HANDOUT
HAIR LOSS

There are many causes of hair loss. Your doctor has diagnosed you with the form called _____. Please refer below to the corresponding circled section.

Tinea capitis—This is a fungus infection. Treatment is only with pills. You must take these as instructed for as long as your doctor has told you. Do not stop the pills as your hair grows back—ask your doctor first. Be sure to keep your doctors appointments to watch for side effects of the drug you are taking. Your hair will grow back completely in 4–6 months.

Alopecia areata—We don't know what causes this disease. The treatment options are limited and hair will grow back, but it may take up to one year.

Pattern baldness—you have inherited this hair loss. Few good treatments are available. Minoxidil works for some. If taking this medicine, follow the instruction carefully. Hair transplants can be done, but these are expensive.

Dermatitis of scalp—Your hair loss is due to a disease of the underlying scalp. Follow your doctors directions and hair will regrow in 3–6 months.

Post partum/post illness telogen effluvium—This fancy name is not important. What you should know is that your hair is going through a natural loss/growth cycle. *DO NOT WORRY.*

Hypothyroidism—we can restore your thyroid hormone, but unfortunately, your hair loss may be permanent. We have no other treatment options.

BENIGN LUMPS AND BUMPS

An enormous variety of benign tumors are found in, under, and on the skin. There exists literally hundreds of benign skin lumps and bumps. Several of these lesions can be derived from each subtype of skin tissue. Tumors of the hair follicle are especially numerous and there are a dozen kinds of sweat gland tumors. Most of these nodules do not require removal. Set conservative criteria for removal. If the tumor is bizarre looking, then most likely the histopathologist will need clinical guidance in arriving at a correct classification. So, be sure to write the clinical appearance, including location, on any biopsy request. Also, if biopsying a lesion, it is cost effective to consult the dermatologist via phone to promote an optimal consultation between primary care and histopathology. This extra effort will allow the biopsy specimen to be reviewed by a pathologist and a dermatologist to ensure the best diagnosis. Keep a tight criteria on choosing which lesions merit biopsy. A very mysterious or unfamiliar lesion is often best managed via immediate referral to your dermatologist.

A few of the most common lumps and bumps are as follows. Remember, this review of benign tumors addresses only a minute proportion of these lesions.

▶ LUMPS

▶ LIPOMAS

BACKGROUND

Lipomas are familial, benign, fatty tumors of the skin. They usually arise during puberty and rarely increase in size. They are usually at their final dimensions when discovered by the patient; 5% of lipoma patients have multiples of these tumors present, but only a few are atypical. Two atypical lipomas are the vascular angiolipoma and the neural neuroma.

IN THE CLINIC

Lipomas are 1–4 cm in diameter, well-demarcated, subcutaneous lumps. They are smooth or multilobular and rubbery to palpation. They can enlarge to the size of a small melon, but this phenomena is rarely seen. Lipomas rarely lead to any secondary problems and they themselves are fully benign. Almost all lipomas are nonpainful, but some angiolipomas and necrolipomas can be painful if pressure is exerted on them.

DIAGNOSIS AND TREATMENT

The diagnosis of a lipoma is undeniably a clinical one. A thorough history and physical examination are usually sufficient in making the diagnosis of a lipoma. Treatment is not necessary unless and angiolipoma or neurolipoma is intensely painful. Treatment for painful lipomas or for cosmetic reasons is performed via simple excision or by liposuction.

PROGNOSIS

Lipomas consist of separate strands of tissue, many of which are woven into adjacent tissues. Thus, even after thorough excision, these lumps often recur in the same location.

MANAGEMENT

▼ Keep all cases.
▼ Reassure patient.

- No need for treatment.
- If cosmetic desire for removal, simple excision
- Explain lesions often recur after removal.

Send

None.

▶ DERMATOFIBROSIS

BACKGROUND

Dermatofibromas are lesions that can occur at any age, but are more common in females. These small lumps are often the result of an insect bite that was aggravated. They are fully benign, but it is important to distinguish them from melanoma.

IN THE CLINIC

These 10–15 mm diameter nodules are usually dome shaped and occur in the upper dermis. They are skin colored or brown and are firm or rubbery to palpation. If squeezed between the thumb and forefinger, they invaginate or pucker. This phenomena is known as the "dimple sign." Most dermatofibromas occur on the extremities with a predilication for the legs.

DIAGNOSIS AND TREATMENT

The diagnosis of a dermatofibroma is usually clinical. Rarely, a dermatofibroma will mimic a malignant melanoma, thus requiring biopsy. Unfortunately, partial removal often leads to regrowth so full excision may be favored when biopsy is necessary. Otherwise, removal of these lesions is wholly cosmetic.

PROGNOSIS

Simple excision of these lesions can be performed if the patient desires, but such removal may lead to scar formation and recurrence is common. These results are not a good bargain in treating a benign lesion.

MANAGEMENT

▼ Keep all cases.
▼ Differentiate clinically from melanoma
▼ Reassure patient
▼ Full, simple excision if:
   1. Biopsy necessary
   2. Cosmetic desire

▶ SEBACEOUS CYST

BACKGROUND

Also known as wens or epidermoid cysts, these lumps are the most common skin cyst seen. They arise from the epidermis and are filled with keratin and lipid. These lesions can occur in any age group or sex and have no malignant potential.

IN THE CLINIC

These lesions are multilobular "bag-like" nodules 1–6 cm in diameter. They usually appear skin colored or slightly white in color and have a smooth surface texture. The cyst wall is thin, thus they are easily traumatized by the patient. If trauma occurs, they can appear inflamed and tender. They may even be the seat for the development of a caruncle.

Often times, a central pore can be seen at the apex of the nodule from which a rancid smelling cheese-like material may be easily expressed. When palpated, a very well-defined, encapsulated nodule is felt deep within the skin or even deeper into subcutaneous margin. Smaller lesions are firmer and often shallow and are often distributed where there are glands, for instance, on the upper trunk, neck, face and scalp.

Epidermoid cysts will enlarge, shrink, and change character frequently. They may spontaneously rupture or rupture secondary to chronic irritation from the patient. In this case, severe inflammation may result and secondary pyodermas may subsequently develop.

DIAGNOSIS AND TREATMENT

The diagnosis of epidermoid cysts is clinical. They differ from lipomas in their encapsulated nature and feel on palpation. Confirmation of the diagnosis can be made by expression of the typical white, pussy material. A simple stab incision should produce a mass of semi-solid cheese-like material on expression. If asymptomatic, these cysts require no treatment. If removal is desired due to repeated trauma or for cosmetic reasons, it can be accomplished via large elliptical excision in the usual surgical manner. Another option includes initial incision and complete drainage after which the cyst shrinks over 1–2 weeks and then can be removed via elliptical excision. If the lesions are inflamed, systemic antibiotics with I&D and hot packs/soaks should be used. Removal of the lesion in such a situation should not be carried out until inflammation has fully resolved.

MANAGEMENT

▼ Keep all cases.
▼ If cosmetic removal desired
▼ Wide elliptical excision
▼ I&D with wide elliptical excision 1–2 weeks later
▼ If inflamed:

Systemic antibiotics (Keflex, Duricef) 500 mg 3 times daily for 1–2 weeks

After oral antibiotics I&D lesions

Hot packs/soaks as needed

ONLY attempt excision when inflammation is resolved.

Send

Few cases that location requires expert cosmetic results (face, genitals)

▶ BUMPS

▶ CHERRY ANGIOMA

BACKGROUND

These vascular lesions first appear in middle adulthood and become more common as the patient ages. They are fully benign with no malignant potential. Their concern is limited to cosmetic appearance only.

IN THE CLINIC

These small superficial lesions occur as dome shaped papules. They vary from pink to red to violet in color and range in size from 2–8 mm. The lesions are not purpuric, but due to the fibrous nature of the involved vessels, they are poorly blanchable. If the lesions are palpated, they are very soft and easily compressed. They can thrombose and their overlying roof is moderately fragile. This thin epidermis may be easily traumatized and result in bleeding. Cherry angiomas are most numerous on the upper trunk, including the chest and back.

DIAGNOSIS AND TREATMENT

The diagnosis is purely clinical. Due to the fully benign and usually asymptomatic character of cherry angiomas, they rarely need treatment. If a patient desires cosmetic removal, it is best performed via light electrosurgery or punch biopsy.

PROGNOSIS

The former gives a slightly better result, but usually requires referral to a specialist. Punch biopsy may leave a tiny scar, but the result is quite acceptable. Once removed, a lesion will not recur. But remember, cherry angiomas increase in number with age. Thus, new lesions may appear solely due to the nature of this skin lesion.

MANAGEMENT

▼ Keep all cases unless desire light electrosurgery.
▼ Reassure patient.

▼ Patient education.

▼ If utilizing punch biopsy for cosmetic removal, no need to send specimen for pathology.

Send

For light electrosurgery (if desired) for cosmetic removal.

▶ MOLLUSCUM CONTAGIOSUM

BACKGROUND

These small skin lesions are seen in children and adults. In the later, they are almost always sexually transmitted. Molluscum are caused by 2 different DNA viruses of the pox virus group. The virus is capable of spreading easily on the non-immune patient via autoinoculation and to others via any close contact. Viral particles are inoculated into the epidermis as a result of cutaneous trauma during close contact. Incubation is from 1–2 months, then explosive growth for several weeks followed by relative stability until they spontaneously resolve 12–24 months later.

IN THE CLINIC

These very superficial lesions are highly distinctive, 2–10 mm diameter papules. Their color ranges from skin colored to almost transparent to near white to tan or dark brown. 25% of lesions have central umbilication. They may occur anywhere, but are most frequently found on the face, arms, and trunk in children, and the lower abdomen, inner thighs, and genitalia in adults. They are almost always numerous and found distributed in a vaguely clustered pattern. Molluscum are usually non-pruritic and almost always asymptomatic.

DIAGNOSIS AND TREATMENT

The diagnosis of molluscum contagiosum is usually clinical. Often, a white globule of viral protein can be extruded from the central portion of the lesion. Biopsy is rarely necessary, but can be performed if the diagnosis is questioned.

PROGNOSIS

Molluscum contagiosum is harmless and will spontaneously remit if left alone. It can be treated to prevent possible spread. Treatment is easiest if performed with cryotherapy for 10–15 seconds. Retreatment is rarely needed and scarring almost never results. Light electrocautery is effective as well, but usually requires referral to a specialist. There is no benefit of light electrotherapy over cryotherapy.

MANAGEMENT

▼ Keep all cases.

▼ Biopsy only if questionable diagnosis.

▼ Treatment is not necessary, these lesions will spontaneously remit.

▼ Patient education.

▼ If cosmetic desire:

Cryotherapy 10–15 seconds, no need to retreat

Send

For cosmetic removal via light electrotherapy.

▶ BACTERIAL FOLLICULITIS

BACKGROUND

These lesions usually represent a superficial infection of the hair follicle with S. aureus. They are most commonly associated with skin trauma as an inciting event. The lesions arise and may last weeks. Certain factors increase the risk of developing folliculitis. These include shaving, hot tub use, and frequent contact with mineral oils.

IN THE CLINIC

These skin lesions are small 1–2 mm diameter pustules that are yellow-grey in color and surrounded by a narrow ring of erythema. They are usually dome shaped, but if a hair is present they will be pointed. They are discrete, occur a few at a time, and *do not cluster*. Commonly affected areas include the face, scalp, and legs if the bacterial insult is S. aureus. Hot tub folliculitis involves a pseudomonal aeruginosa etiology and lesions are usually on the trunk. Folliculitis is not associated with fever or lymphadenopathy.

DIAGNOSIS AND TREATMENT

The diagnosis of folliculitis is usually clinical. A gram stain should show g(+) cocci in clusters in the majority of cases. A bacterial culture is diagnostic but very rarely necessary. Treatment of bacterial folliculitis depends on the number of actual lesions. If one or two lesions present topical antibiotics applied two times daily are usually effective. If more than two pustules, it is more effective. If more than two pustules, it is more efficient and effective to place the patient on oral anti-staphylococcal antibiotics. For example, oral Keflex (250–500 mg) four times daily for 7–10 days. Untreated pustules will spontaneously resolve without treatment in about 7 days as well. But usually, as one lesion heals itself, another forms nearby.

PROGNOSIS

The prognosis for bacterial folliculitis is good. Treated lesions usually heal within 10 days and rarely involve scarring. On rare occasion, bacterial folliculitis can lead to cellulitis or furuncularis.

MANAGEMENT

▼ Keep all cases.

▼ Gram stain or culture if questionable bacterial etiology.

▼ If < 2 lesions, topical antibiotics two times daily for 7–10 days.

▼ If > 2 lesions, oral anti-staph antibiotics (ex., Keflex [250–500 mg] four times daily for 7–10 days)

▶ SEBORRHEIC KERATOSIS

BACKGROUND

These benign skin lesions begin to appear after age 30 and proliferate as aging continues. The lesions themselves have no malignant potential and sunlight exposure plays no role in their development. There is believed to be a genetic predisposition in terms of the age of onset and number of these lesions present. There may be an autosomal dominant pattern of inheritance.

IN THE CLINIC

These flat-topped papules start as small light brown 1–3 mm diameter lesions. Over time, they enlarge in diameter to form 10–20 mm plaques, which are dark brown in color. All lesions are well demarcated from surrounding skin. Their surface has a "greasy" or "stuck on" appearance typical of seborrheic keratosis. If taken in cross-section, they appear "square-shouldered." The lesions are discrete and do no cluster. They are most common on the trunk, but are also seen on the face and proximal upper extremities.

DIAGNOSIS AND TREATMENT / IV PROGNOSIS

The diagnosis is usually clinical and easily made. Unfortunately, seborrheic keratoses may resemble actinic keratoses or melanoma, in which case, shave biopsy is warranted for diagnosis. These can be quickly and easily performed in the primary care clinic. Seborrheic keratoses do not require treatment due to their benign nature. But, many patients ask for their removal for cosmetic reasons. This removal is easily performed in the primary care setting with shave biopsy or cryotherapy (10–15 seconds). Light electrosurgery is also effective, but often requires referral to a specialist. Once treated, these lesions rarely recur in the same location. Remember that with age, they increase in number. So, treating one lesion will not keep new lesions from developing at different locations.

MANAGEMENT

▼ Keep all cases unless light electrosurgery for removal.
▼ Remove for cosmetic reasons only via:
   1. Shave biopsy
   2. Cryotherapy (10–15 seconds)
▼ Biopsy if questionable diagnosis via shave biopsy.

Send

If cosmetic removal desired with light electrosurgery.

PEARLS AND PITFALLS

▼ Lipomas and dermatofibromas can recur after removal.

▼ Dermatofibromas are felt to develop from aggravated insect bites.

▼ Best to treat sebaceous cysts with 1–2 week course of antibiotics *before* attempting wide elliptical excision.

▼ Cherry angiomas and seborrheic keratosis increase in number as the patient ages.

▼ Molluscum contagiosum in adult is a sexually transmitted disease.

▼ Most bacterial folliculitis is due to staph aureus. Hot tub folliculitis is due to pseudomonas aeruginosa.

CASE 6.3

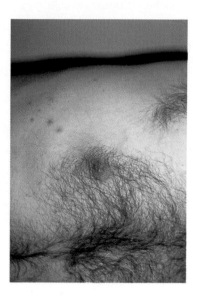

S: A 23-year-old male actor presents to your clinic in Los Angeles, California with complaints of a bumpy rash on his lower torso and legs bilaterally. He states that the rash has been present for 1 day and is worrisome to him. He is the lead character in a B rated film that is currently in production and requires him to be shirtless in many scenes. He won't be able to perform the required work until the rash clears up. He denies any itching or pain associated. He admits to never having had such a rash in the past. He denies any pertinent past medical history and is otherwise feeling well. He reveals that, in fact, his acting career has really taken off lately allowing him to buy a large condominium with a hot tub. He states he wants to invite you and your staff to his place for a big celebration and "hot tub" party in 2 weeks if you would just clear up his rash. Further questioning reveals that he had a similar party 2 days prior which he felt was quite successful.

O: A pleasant young man who is affable and cooperative to examination.

Skin—Multiple, small (1–2mm diameter), well-demarcated, discrete greyish pustules with a thin border of erythema around the margins are seen widely scattered over the patients trunk and lower extremities. The lesions are numerous and vary from dome shaped to pointed in appearance. The skin is otherwise WNL.

The rest of the examination is unremarkable.

A: Hot tub folliculitis.

P: Oral anti-pseudomonas antibiotic for 7 days. Vinegar soaks will speed healing.

Advise of source and recommend a thorough cleaning of his new hot tub prior to the planned party.

PATIENT EDUCATION HANDOUT
LUMPS AND BUMPS

The skin lesion you have been diagnosed with *is not a cancer* and has no chance of developing into a cancer.

The skin lesion you have is called a _____.

Below are some specifics on your skin lesion:

▶ BITES AND STINGS

BACKGROUND

Many insects, spiders, and snakes thrive in our environment. These creatures are often responsible for stings/bites to patients and can lead to skin changes at the site of the injury as well as generalized rashes in some cases. This text will not attempt to give detail on all such bites/stings for the breadth of the subject is vast. Highlights are given below—we recommend "Arthropods and Human Skin" by John O'Donal Alexander; Springer-Varlag 1984 Berlin, for a comprehensive text on insects, spiders, and their stings. For snakes use current regional literature, because snake bites are very different in various parts of the country. Also, this chapter is organized via type of inciting creature rather than the typical organizations of previous chapters.

IN THE CLINIC

Common insect bites/stings are caused by bees, wasps, hornets, mites, chiggers, mosquitos, fleas, gnats, and lice to name a few.

DIAGNOSIS AND TREATMENT

Scabies

Scabies is a quite common infestation which often leads to a characteristic, pruritic rash. This infestation was thoroughly reviewed in its own section in chapter 7. Please see these pages for detail in regards to scabies and its rash.

Bees, Wasps, Hornets

The most common serious stings are by bees, wasps, or hornets. These insects are truly aggressive, often attack in swarms, and we can see cases of multiple bites. These stings can become disabling especially in children. These stings are manifested clinically by immediate pain and quick swelling and erythema at the injured site. Edema can be severe enough as to distort regular anatomical features—especially facial features. Most of these stings have associated localized pruritus which may last 7–10 days. In addition, there may be sudden symmetrical mild swelling of the eyelids, lips, hands, and feet. This edema is *not* a sign of anaphylaxis but rather a disseminated reaction to the insect sting. If the sting is causing anaphylaxis the patient will manifest severe, generalized skin, urticaria or angioedema, will vary in degrees of progression, mental confusion, hypotension, and comprise of the airway.

Treatment of mild to moderate stings that remain localized or with dissemination only is add pack application to the injured site every 1 hour, rest, oral antihistamines immediately with redosing every 6–8 hours after the sting. NSAID's are the best form of analgesia to aid in pain relief.

If a patient is experiencing anaphylaxis they should be treated emergently with airway maintenance, IV access, subcutaneous 1:1000 epinephrine (0.4 cc in adults) in the upper chest and at site of sting, and prompt, calm transport to an emergency room. Every clinic should have a previously arranged plan such as this one for managing anaphylaxis. These patients usually respond well to simple subcutaneous epinephrine treatment and the individual should be advised to have an epi-pen handy in the future and should be instructed on its use in case a repeat sting occurs.

Other Insects

Those bites by chiggers, mosquitos, fleas and gnats are almost always benign. Occasionally we see local edema. The principle goal in uncomplicated lesions is to relieve any associated pruritus as to prevent excoriation and possible secondary pyoderma. Most patients handle these lesions at home with topical steroid creams available over the counter. If the pruritus is severe, cold packs, oral antihistamines, and rest will cure the majority of these bites. Reducing the itch allows for prompt healing and reduces the likelihood of a pyoderma developing. Remind the patient to look for increase in redness, pain, edema and any exudate, or presence of tender local lymph nodes. These are signs of possible pyoderma and these patients need to be seen in the clinic to determine if an oral anti-staphloccol antibiotic is necessary. Very infrequently do insect bites other than those by bees, wasps, and hornets lead to anaphylaxis.

Snakes

The two most frequently seen venomous snake bites in the U.S. are those inflicted by the copperhead and the rattlesnake. Other snakes also cause venomous bites and the type of snake, its behavior, and its venom differ region to region. Each local medical group must know their own snakes well to manage such bites correctly. Rare or pet snakes often pose a unique problem. In such situations you often must rely on history to determine the type of snakebite with which you are dealing. The most popular means by which people are bitten by snakes is the actual physical picking up of these reptiles. If proper clothing and footwear is worn in snake prone areas, individuals use good wood craft skills, and snakes are not handled, bites are uncommon. Thus, prevention is key in the management of snake bites.

When examining skin that is suspected of being snake-bite, look for characteristic findings. First attempt to visualize any puncture marks. If two are seen, this indicates the lesions are sustained from a creatures fangs. Carefully measure the distance between these puncture wounds. Fang spacing is an indicator of the size of the snake and its potential for serious envenomation. If the snake is of a nonvenomous variety, they have rows of teeth without fangs and the bite displays a grooved appearance rather than two-spaced punctures.

If a snake is of venomous nature, its bite can be a serious medical emergency. If you feel a patient has been bitten by a venomous snake, they should be sent directly to an emergency room. Most emergency settings have protocols available on how to manage a bite by a local venomous snake. Most patients are admitted for at least 24 hours of observation after emergency treatment is rendered. Antivenom is a hazardous substance and should be used only by those physicians well versed in its use.

A snake bite that displays a grooved change in the skin is, as previously mentioned, indicative of a nonvenomous creature. Such findings are reassuring. Such snake bites need no dermatological referral. They are best handled by simple proper wound care.

Spiders

We often see patients in the clinic who present with concern over a spider bite. The vast majority of these wounds are small with mild erythema, edema, and pain or pruritus. These bites are handled best with local wound care and prevention of possible secondary pyoderma. Some spiders are more venomous than others. But even these "more dangerous" varieties rarely cause more than a painful bite with the above changes and possible a *small* amount of necrosis. These bites appear quite similar to an uncomplicated bee, wasp, or hornet sting. Management of these sites is the same as other spider bites.

Really, only two spiders in the U.S. are of medical importance, the black widow and the brown recluse. The black widow spider imports a neurotoxin that incites a hyper-reactivity of the nervous system that leads to symptoms including confusion and hallucination. The brown recluse imports a toxic necrolysin that can produce a very large areas of necrosis and skin ulceration. The average wound is 2.0 cm in diameter. This spider's toxic bite can also cause sudden, severe systemic hemolysis with associated anuria. These severe reactions are seen mainly in children who have been bitten by a brown recluse spider. If a patient presents with a large area of local skin ulceration and necrosis, and a spider bite is suspected as the possible etiology, immediate phone consultation with a dermatologist may prove helpful. The key concern is to not overlook other possible etiologies of the wound such as a primary infection (example: necrotizing, fasciitis). A severe bacterial infection may look like a spider bite. Be cautious—Spider bites may produce brief fever and leukocytosis which lead to a close infectious mimic. But, in contrast, spider bites never cause lymphadenopathy early as do primary infections.

All suspected black widow bites need to be watched closely for possible neurologic sequela. If such nervous system symptoms develop the patient requires a neurological consult, hospitalization, and further inpatient treatment. A brown recluse bite that measures less than 2 cm in diameter is appropriately handled in the primary care setting with close observation and proper wound care. Any skin changes subsequent to a brown recluse spider bite that measure greater than 2 cm in diameter are best handled by dermatological referral. These wounds can be quite serious and the toxic potential of the bite can lead to systemic hemolysis and possible subsequent renal failure and anuria. If you have an interest in the bites of these spiders and are adapt at handling their care, a referral need not be performed.

MANAGEMENT

To Manage

▼ Keep:

All ordinary insects, bees, wasps, hornet stings.

Any nonvenomous snake bites

Any spider bites with or without necrosis that measures < 2 cm in diameter.

▼ Treat—bees/wasps/hornets

Local cold pack application

Oral antihistamines PRN pruritus

Any sign of secondary pyoderma

Anaphylactic reactions with:

1. Airway maintenance
2. Subcutaneous 1:1000 epinephrine 0.44 cc at wound site and 0.4 cc in skin of chest.
3. Prompt transport to ER by ambulance
4. IV access if available

▼ Common insect bites:

Cold packs locally

Oral antihistamines PRN pruritus

Topical OTC corticosteroid creams/ointments

Any sign of secondary pyoderma

▼ Snake bites (nonvenomous)

Analgesics (NSAID; most effective)

Local wound care

▼ Spider bites < 2 cm diameter

Same as common insect bites above.

Send

▼ All anaphylactic reactions for prompt ER care after establishing airway, IV, and administering subcutaneous epinephrine 1:1000— 0.4cc in skin of chest and 0.4 cc at site of bite/sting.

▼ Any snake bite suspected to be venomous to ER.

▼ All necrotizing spider bites > 2 cm in diameter.

PROGNOSIS

With expert care and management as outlined in the previous sections of this chapter, most bites and stings have a very good prognosis. Any necrotizing spider bite or bite/sting that develops a large secondary pyoderma has the potential to leave a subsequent scar.

PEARLS AND PITFALLS

▼ Reassuring the patient about bites that are not serious is a key portion of managing all bites and stings.

▼ Always prescribes epi-pens to any patient with a history of anaphylaxic reactions. Have them keep these devices available at
home, school, day care, etc.

▼ Advise of topical insect repellents that these are effective. Herbal
remedies or various vitamins have never been proven to serve as
possible aids in repelling insects.

▼ Chart any history of allergic bite/sting reaction.

CASE 6.4

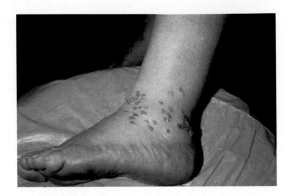

S: A 15-year-old male presents to your clinic one summer morning with complaints of a 3-day history of "insect bites" on his legs. The bites are quite itchy. and he has been scratching them according to his mother who has accompanied him on this visit. They have been putting antibiotic ointment on the wounds but it has not changed them in any manner. Further questioning reveals that the young man mows lawns for his summer job and spends 8–10 hours/day on both riding and push mowers. He commonly wears shorts, ankle socks, and shoes while working.

O: A Pleasant, young man.

Skin: Face, back, chest demonstrate a mild sunburn without blisters. Legs bilaterally with numerous (25 erythematosus, excoriated papules 3–5 mm in diameter. Located proximal to his ankle sock line and sitral to his tibial tuberosity. The lesions are not warm, under or exudative. No scale, fissuring or pustules seen. No lesions on feet, ankles. Rest of skin and physical examination is WNR.

A: Insect bites; multiple—probable chiggers.

P: Continue to use topical antibiotic to reduce chance of secondary pyoderma.

Add topical OTC corticosteroid cream 1 or 2% Hydrocortisone cream BID to areas of bites to reduce itch.

If topical steroid not sufficient to relieve itch, and avoid scratching, add oral antihistamine 25–50mg every 8 hours.

Educate on pyoderma and have them call if any signs/symptoms of such a skin infection develops.

Wear knee-high socks and pants when cutting lawns to prevent such bites.

PATIENT EDUCATION HANDOUT
BITES AND STINGS

Your bite is most likely from a _____.

Follow the below directions as circled below to care for this bite:

A. Place cold packs (wet or dry) on area of bite. Do this for 15 min. Every 1–2 hours until improved.
B. Ibuprofen dose—_____ for any pain.
C. You may use a topical over the counter steroid cream $1/2\%$–2% two to three times a day for itching.
D. If itching is severe, you may use an oral antihistamine. We suggest: _____.

If the area bitten becomes more red, swollen, tender, warm or any pus develops, phone your doctor right away to let them know. These are signs of possible infection.

▶ MELANOMA

BACKGROUND

Cutaneous melanoma is a malignancy of the melanocytes of the skin and mucous membrane. This skin cancer has become a prime medical concern to many patients. Individuals are becoming more aware of melanoma due to heightened attention in television and print-journalism. Patients really worry about this cancer. They have been exposed to some of the following frightening data.

Melanoma is the most rapidly increasing form of cancer in the white-skinned populations. It is the second most common form of cancer in men aged 30–49. It is a disease whose primary form predominately affects young and middle aged persons; 80% of melanoma is caused by exposure to sunlight—most especially a history of sunburn. Also, mortality rates from primary melanoma have been increasing 1% per year in women and 3% per year in men. Such statistics have led anxious patients to their physicians to analyze certain skin pigmentations they fear may be melanoma.

Even though the number of individuals dying from melanoma is becoming a lesser percentage of overall deaths in this country, those patients diagnosed with melanoma are experiencing increasing 5 year and 10-year survival rates. This phenomena can be directly linked to early detection and diagnosis of these pigmented lesions. The general concern the patient population has with melanoma can be used to the physicians advantage when it comes to getting patients into the clinic for regular skin checks and educating them about melanoma.

IN THE CLINIC

Dealing with melanoma in the clinic setting is most easily approached by a 3-pronged attached method. The first challenge is to recognize those patients who are at high risk for developing the disease. The second tactic is learning how to perform a screening mole check and finding a way to incorporate it into your standard screening physical examination. Thirdly, the physician must learn to be adapt at recognizing melanoma and managing it quickly and correctly. In the managed care setting, routine biopsy of "any odd" mole is no longer acceptable. The cost of biopsy and the subsequent associated histopathology is quite high. Physicians in such capitated plans need to learn to recognize suspicious moles and biopsy only those they find concerning rather than taking off any mole the patient is worried over.

First, let us approach the recognition of a high risk patient. The single greatest risk factor for melanoma is a family history of melanoma. Always ask about melanoma when covering the patients family history during your screening health maintenance examination. About 10% of melanoma has a positive family history. It is best the mode of inheritance may be reautosomal dominant. A family history of basal cell and squamous cell skin cancer also increases a patients risk for developing melanoma. Other risk factors include fair-skin with predisposition to sunburn, the present of numerous common moles, excessive sunlight exposure, and the presence of any atypical moles. Melanoma is quite rare in childhood unless the patient is afflicted with a large congenital melanocytic nevus. Which is considered a risk factor for melanoma in this age group. Black and dark skinned individuals can develop melanoma but are at a four-fold less risk of doing so. The actual etiology behind the development of melanoma in these patients is not yet known.

Now that we know who is at risk to develop melanoma we must learn how to screen a patient for this skin cancer. Patients will either come to the office with concern over a specific mole or to have you look at their skin in general for any peculiar moles. These are not the only patients on whom you perform a "mole-check." Such skin cancer screening needs to be incorporated into each individual's routine examination. Either annually for low risk individuals or every 6 months for any patients with high risk factors as mentioned above. When examining the skin be certain you have good light and always use dermatoscopy or a 5x magnifying lens. It is quite feasible to draw a detailed "map" of any nevus that appears borderline or questionable. These maps can be used again when reexamining this group of nevi for changes—optimally every 60–120 days. Frequent examination allows for a cost-effective analysis of these moles in regards to the crucial issue of disorderly change over time. These moles are best handled collaboratively with a dermatologist. Often a phone consultation will do. Collaborative efforts and frequent, thorough examination cuts back on the time and cost of unnecessary biopsy while addressing the patients concerns. Also, always stress the importance of patients performing self-skin examinations on a routine basis. These areas not easily checked on one's own body can be examined routinely by a family member.

The third important concept in the approach of melanoma is recognizing a highly suspicious lesion and handling the assumed melanoma in an appropriate fashion. Remember that this skin cancer is curable and curability depends upon early recognition and removal. Only 15–20% of melanoma arises from preexisting nevi (see nevus section 7.5). The rest of these skin cancers arise de novo from normal appearing skin. Thus, always ask about new or fast growing/changing lesions. Remember most individuals should have little change in their moles after age 25. The exception is pregnancy, and we have approached this topic in the nevus section previously.

Melanoma spreads horizontally at first then progresses to a vertically spreading phase from which it begins regional lymph node infiltration and metastasis. The prognosis is far better if the lesion is caught during the period of horizontal spread. Different forms of melanoma remain in this radial phase for differing amounts of time depending on the form of melanoma that is present. But all forms of melanoma are best prognostically if detected early in the horizontal or radial phase for it is during this time that the tumor is "thin." As the cancer grows vertically and becomes thicker, the prognosis worsens. An A type melanoma < 1.0 mm in depth has a 10-year survival rate of 90%. A lesion > 4.0mm in depth has only a 50% 5-year survival rate. Thus, we want to catch the cancer as early as possible before it begins to grow deeper and worsen the disease prognosis.

Now lets look at how to differentiate a melanoma from a nevus. The A-B-C-D criteria should always be applied. These rules are the basis of melanoma diagnosis described by most textbooks and we feel are most suitable in the managed care setting as well. ABCD refers to *A*symmetry, *B*order irregularities, *C*olor, and *D*iameter.

> Asymmetry: Draw a line through the center of the lesion. Are the two sides mirror images or is one-half unlike the other half. Moles are usually symmetrical while melanoma is usually asymmetric.
>
> Border: Moles have clean, tidy, well-circumscribed edges. Melanoma is characterized by pseudopods, islands, and/or outcroppings of pigment.
>
> Color: Melanoma displays variation in the color of the lesion itself. There may be shading or black tan and brown colors, or a mixture of colors from one area to another. Special concern should be given to dots of red, white, blue or pitch black.
>
> Diameter: Primarily look at *change* in size. Melanoma change in

size and the diameter will increase. Moles almost always stay the same size after they fully develop (~ age 25). Although melanoma can be any size, look very closely at those lesions > 6mm diameter.

We have placed a card made by the American Academy of Dermatology (AAD) for melanoma screening in the back cover of this book for your use.

Unfortunately, melanoma screening by the ABCD criteria is not perfect. These guidelines are so broad they include a great number of normal nevi, seborrheic keratosis, vascular spots and pyogenic granulomas. If we were to apply the ABCD rules to pubertal children, a vast number of benign nevi would be removed due to the rapid change/growth of such lesions during this period of life. In patients over age 50 an-old nevus will fibrosis and can cause an acute size change. Pregnancy can lead to darkening of benign nevi and may cause a nevus to appear "new." Folliculitis can cause a nevus to become tender or change color. Thus, use these A-B-C-D rules to screen for concerning lesions. *Then* look further at those moles that are concerning. If the patient is < 25 years old, has only a few nevi total, and is not in a high risk category, a skin map can be employed as earlier outlined.

If you have concerns or questions, consultation via phone or a single visit referral to the collaborating dermatologist is very helpful. Often the specialist will reaffirm your decision to not biopsy and watch closely. This technique is made even easier with telemedicine or computer link. If you have telemedicine capabilities, work out a method of consultation via this modality. All of these aforementioned "second opinion" options are much cheaper and less time consuming than biopsy and enable patient reassurance.

DIAGNOSIS AND TREATMENT

Most melanoma are discovered in the clinical setting as outlined in the previous section. A lesion that is highly suspicious should always be biopsied during the same clinical visit. Giving a patient a "follow-up" visit-even within a week allows for the possibility of noncompliance in lesion removal. Perform a punch biopsy on lesions that permit removal of 1–2mm normal appearing tissue bordering the pigmented lesion. If the suspect lesion is too large to permit effective punch biopsy, an incisional biopsy may be performed. We have given a detailed account of how to properly perform a punch biopsy in this chapter.

If possible, collaborate with the dermatologist when sending a suspected melanoma biopsy for dermatopathology. Often the pathologist inspecting your biopsy is not as well versed on skin pathology as is the dermatologist. Review of the dermatopathology by a dermatologist is fruitful in procuring the appropriate diagnosis. Any lesion that is melanoma on biopsy requires referral to a dermatologist for further treatment. This additional therapy may include further excision, exploration of lymph nodes if suspect, and radiation therapy. Thus, treatment is via referral. The primary care physician should again collaborate with the speciality to enable return to the primary care clinic for maintenance after treatment and continued close screening for any new suspicious lesions.

MANAGEMENT

To Manage

▼ Keep all patients for screening mole checks.

1. Every 12 months if no risk factors
2. Every 6 months if risk factors present

▼ Any mildly suspicious lesions

1. Keep "skin map" and *watch for change.*
2. Re-check every 60 to 120 days

▼ Biopsy all highly suspicious lesions.

1. Best if biopsy during same visit as diagnosis.
2. Punch biopsy if possible with 1–2 cm border of normal tissue.
3. Excisional biopsy for all lesions too large to punch biopsy effectively.

▼ Those patients diagnosed with melanoma *after* referral for that lesion. Continue skin checks—now every 6 months, skin maps if indicated, and biopsies where indicated.

▼ Patient education on melanoma, risk factors, prognosis, and the importance of self-examination on regular basis.

Send

▼ Biopsy proven melanoma for treatment ASAP.

▼ Any lesion that is questionable for consultation (cheaper and less invasive than biopsy).

PROGNOSIS

A variety of prognostic data was given earlier in this chapter. Again, the prognosis of this deadly skin cancer is dependent on the thickness of the biopsied lesion. Deeper lesions have allowed more time for possible lymph node involvement and metastatic spread. The *overall* 5-year survival rate for all melanomas is about 80%. Once lesions have metastasized the chance for cure is dismal. Thus, *early diagnosis* is key in the prognosis of melanoma.

PEARLS AND PITFALLS

Consult your dermatologist over the phone when sending a biopsy. They can review the dermatopathology and aid in proper diagnosis.

If you remove a mole and miss part of it—it may reoccur. Biopsy of the reoccurring mole will demonstrate marked atypical changes. Be certain to note a specimen is a rebiopsy on the pathology form.

When screening look at *all of the skin.* Pay particular attention to the back, shoulders, vulva, anus, mouth, scalp and legs. In dark skinned patients, look closely at the palms and soles.

Never remove a mole without sending it for pathological confirmation. If you are concerned enough that you want to remove the lesion, then it should be sent for histopathologic study.

If removing a pigmented lesion for cosmetic reasons, explain to the patient that all of these are sent to pathology for microscopic diagnosis. Patients must incur the expense of removal and pathology if the lesion is being excised for cosmetic reasons only—make certain they are aware of this cost before proceeding. Often times they will decide that the $225 mole on their left shoulder is not so unattractive after all.

CASE 6.5

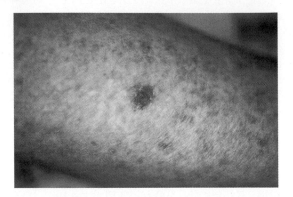

S: A 32-year-old white female, Megin O'Malley, presents to your clinic in Boston for a routine skin check. The O'Malleys are well known to your practice. You diagnosed Megan's aunt with melanoma about 3 months ago. This diagnosis promoted Megan's visit today. The blue-eyed redhead has just returned from a week at the families vacation home on Cape cod and admits to frequent sunburn and rare tanning. She does not routinely check her own skin and complains of no lesions of concern.

O: A well-nourished young female. *Skin*—fair complexion with mild sunburn. Multiple brown spots are widely scattered over nose, cheeks, shoulders and chest. A few (total = 6) well-demarcated light brown plaques 2–4 mm in diameter on shoulder, back, chest – all with uniform pigmentation and symmetry. Just superior medially to the right knee is a 5-mm diameter dark brown plaque with a blue-grey hue. The color is variegated. There is a small (.5 mm diameter) plaque that is tender to palpation at about 2:00. The lesion is asymmetrical with an irregular, notched border. Megan states the lesion has been present for 1 or 2 years; she states it is larger now that she looks closely at it then she remembers it being. The skin has no other remarkable findings.

A: Possible melanoma right thigh; multiple benign solar lentigo and ephelides shoulders, back and chest; numerous lentigo.

P: Patient is in high risk category due to her family history of melanoma. You perform a 6-mm punch biopsy of the lesion and send it for pathology. Phone collaboration with the dermatologist on the dermatopathology is performed. The lesion is determined to be a superficial spreading melanoma with 1 mm of depth (Breslow). Patient is referred to the dermatologist for complete management of this melanoma with instructions to continue with 6-month visits to check skin. Patient education provided as well.

PATIENT EDUCATION HANDOUT
MELANOMA

Your physician has taken a mole from your skin that has been diagnosed as a melanoma.

You will be referred to a dermatologist for further treatment of this skin cancer.

Melanoma is a skin cancer. Different types of melanoma have different prognosis or outcomes. Ask your physician to explain what type of melanoma you have and how serious it is.

Continue to check your skin with a family member's help on a monthly basis.

Stress the importance of regular skin exams to your family—your having this skin cancer increases the chance they might develop one as well.

Continue to see your physician regularly for skin checks—*every 6 months*. See him/her immediately if you see a mole that worries you.

Use the A-B-C-D criteria on the card provided to look for moles that need to be checked by your doctor.

▶ NAIL DISEASE AND DEFORMITY

BACKGROUND

The normal nail forms as a hard plate arising from specialized epithelial cells. The hard nail plate is made up of Keratin and begins deep to the proximal nail fold. It extends out over the soft tissue nail bed and provides the hard nail plate with support. This hard nail plate overlying the soft tissue nail bed is the pink colored portion of the nail, except the most proximal part, which is white, crescent shaped and termed the lunula. The cuticle is the soft tissue that joins the proximal and lateral nail folds to the nail plate. The most distal portion of the hard nail plate is white in color due to light refraction under the free edge.

Many nail diseases and systemic illnesses demonstrate changes to one or more portions of the normal nail. It often takes weeks for the diseased nail matrix to be visualized. This phenomena occurs because changes can only be seen once the damaged portion of the nail grows out from under the proximal nail fold. This "grow-out-lag" phenomena also causes treated nails to require approximately 3 months to fully grow out and be replaced by a normal nail.

In this chapter, we will review a few of the most common nail dystrophies and those diseases which may clinically manifest with nail changes. These diseases include subungual hematoma, ingrown nail, psoriasis, onychomycosis, oncolysis, Beau's grooves, periungual warts, clubbing, herpetic whitlow, paronychia, splinter hemorrhages, tumors, and severe systemic illness.

DIAGNOSIS AND TREATMENT

Subungual Hematoma—Macro trauma or repetitive micro trauma to the tips of the digits can lead to the formation of blood collection under the hard nail plate. These resulting subungual hematomas can be quite painful and if large enough will lead to loss of the overlying hard nail plate.

If a subungual hematoma is large enough it can be exquisitely painful. Pain is best relieved via draining the hematoma with electrocautery. Pain is significantly reduced after this procedure. Unfortunately, even if drained, the subungual hematoma may have caused enough underlying nail matrix damage to lead to deformity or loss of the hard nail plate. A new nail will regrow. But, if damage to the nail bed was significant, the newly formed nail may be deformed in shape as well. Unfortunately, no treatment exists to cure this problem and the patient is left with a chronically deformed nail plate.

Oncolysis—Onycholysis is a separation of the distal nail plate from the nail bed. The resulting nail appears as if the normally white distal edge has progressed proximally into the area that is usually pinkish in color. This separation and its accompanied whitening is often associated with brittleness and distal splintering of the nail. This phenomena is also known as *plumber's nail*.

Onycholysis can have various etiologies, the most common being a candidal infection associated with a wet working environment. Other possible etiologies include hyperthyroidism, trauma, psoriasis, and chemical exposure.

Treatment of oncolysis involves care of the underlying etiology as listed above. If the causative disease is not eliminated, the nail change will persist.

Paronychia—Paronychia may develop secondarily to a candidal or bacterial infection. Candidal associated paronychia are most common and may involve oncolysis as well. Such fungal infections are most commonly associated with prolonged work in a wet environment (housekeeping, bartending, dishwashing).

Clinically, candidal paronychia are chronically erythematous, nonpainful, cool to the touch, and without associate exudate. Diagnosis can be made with a KOH preparation although, obtaining an appropriate specimen is often difficult. If you do decide to KOH a paronychia, remember, a negative result does not rule out a fungal origin. Thus, we feel that paronychia are best diagnosed clinically and without a KOH.

Treatment of candidal paronychia is best approached with topical antifungals specific for yeast. Lotrimin is a good choice. The antifungal should be applied to the involved soft tissue three times daily for approximately two weeks. Leave the affected digit open to the air so as to minimize the moisture in the environment of the affected soft tissue.

Bacterial paronychia are also erythematous, but unlike their candidal cousins, they are extremely painful, edematous, tender and associated with pus. The majority of bacterial paronychia begin when staphylococcus that is indigenous to the intact skin invades the periungual region as a result of trauma. Treatment of these nail infections is via twice daily soaks in warm, soapy water and oral anti staphylococcus antibiotics three times daily for 5–7 days. Although many physicians incise and drain these lesions, such a maneuver is not necessary and need not be performed.

Ingrown Nails—Such a phenomena occurs almost exclusively in the great toenail. It is the most common etiology of bacterial paronychia. The toenail edge is liable to pierce the surrounding soft tissue in situations where toenails have been clipped too short, shoes are too tight, or in sports where sudden stops cause the toenail to be forced proximally.

Treatment of ingrown toenails requires two steps. At the first visit, the free edge of the nail should be lifted and cotton placed under it. The patient should be sent home with instructions to soak in warm water 2–3 times daily and replace the cotton. Also, at the initial visit, place the patient on a 5–7 day course of anti staphylococcal antibiotics three times daily. See the patient back in the office in one week.

At that time, removal of the distal nail lateral plate with a Beaver Blade is one option. Otherwise, surgical removal of the entire lateral nail plate and associated matrix under sterile conditions and local anesthesia can be carried out. The nail should be rechecked one week after surgery to ensure the onset of proper healing. Explain to the patient that the new nail will take approximately three months to grow back out. Also, stress toenail care with clipping horizontally, not clipping too short, and proper shoe wear. Such prevention should limit recurrence of ingrown nails.

Herpetic Whitlow—A paronychial infection may occur secondary to the herpes simplex virus and is then known as a herpetic whitlow. It is often seen in individuals who routinely have their hands exposed to other peoples mouth. This group includes dentists, nurses, and other health care providers.

The lesions resemble a bacterial paronychia with warmth, erythema, edema, and pain. Herpetic whitlow can be differentiated from bacterial paronychia by the usual presence of tiny clustered vesicles on an erythematous base. The lesions will resolve spontaneously in 7–10 days, thus treatment with oral antiviral medication is not necessary. Cool water or Burow's solution soaks in combination with oral analgesics may help reduce the pain of these lesions.

Onychomycosis—This dermatophyte infection of the nail plate is most often caused by Candida or Trichophyton rubrum. It is most often seen in the toenails and older age appears to be a predisposing factor. As one ages, blood flow to the nail becomes less and the nail becomes more susceptible to fungal infections. Usually, infected nails are present at the same time as noninfected nails.

Clinically, the nails appear as one of two abnormalities. The first possible change is a brownish-yellow color to the distal free edge with the associated separation of the nail plate from the nail bed. In the associated space, keratin debris builds up due to subungual hyperkeratosis. The other possible clinical finding is a whitened distal free edge with increased brittleness and roughness of the nail. Oncomycosis closely resembles psoriatic nail changes. Both presentations are treated similarly.

Diagnosis can be clinical only, but is best supported with KOH to help differentiate dermatophyte infection from psoriatic nail changes (please see dermatophyte chapter for specifics on how to perform this test correctly). Treatment of choice is terbinafine 150 mg orally each day for up to 12 weeks. This medication has superb penetrance into the nail matrix to cure the diseased nail. Of course, treatment need not occur. Oncomycosis causes nothing but cosmetic deformity. Often the cost of treatment with an effective oral agent outweighs the cosmetic benefit of therapy. Reassure the patient that the fungal infection is not contagious nor will it be transmitted from nail to nail on a single individual.

Psoriasis—25% of patients with psoriasis have involvement of the nails. Nail changes usually follow the other characteristic lesions. Clinically, the nails may demonstrate oncolysis with underlying subungual keratin build up similar to oncomycosis. In such a situation, a careful history and examination for other psoriatic manifestations and a KOH to rule out dermatophytosis should be performed. Another possible nail change in psoriasis is "oil spots." These lesions are yellow-brown dots that form between the nail bed and the nail plate. The final clinical presentation is "ice pick stippling." This change is manifested as pits on the nail's surface and can enlarge to the point of severe nail dystrophy.

Diagnosis is usually clinical with a KOH if necessary to rule out onychomycosis. Specific treatment of psoriatic nails is debatable. Steroid injections into the nail fold are effective, but can be painful and may lead to nail atrophy. The best method of treatment is to treat the patient's skin psoriasis with UVB phototherapy, PUVA, or methotrexate. These skin treatments will usually lead to resolution of the nail changes as well.

Periungual Warts—Verruca vulgaris often occur at sites of trauma, one of which may be the nail plate. Nail biting, chewing, or repetitive trauma can lead to the formation of these unsightly nail lesions. If large enough, these warts can lead to changes in the nail plate itself. Thus, significant nail dystrophy can occur.

Diagnosis is purely clinical and these lesions are easily differentiated from other possible etiologies of nail dystrophy. Treatment of the periungual warts is by cryotherapy or DNCB as outlined in the chapter on Verrucous Vulgaris. Most often, resolution of the warts is followed by the return of the nail plate to its normal appearance. If the dystrophy is severe and long standing, some degree of nail plate abnormality may persist despite resolution of the wart itself.

Beau's Grooves—These nail changes can follow severe systemic illness, such as malnutrition, MI, PE, shock. They form as a result of lowered protein synthesis during such stresses which leads to cessation of nail growth. The grooves are seen as 1–2 mm wide horizontal depressions that extend from one edge of the nail plate to the other. All nails are affected simultaneously. Changes are not seen until 2–3 weeks after the physiologic stressor due to their initial occurrence in the nail matrix. It takes this much time for the grooved nail to grow out to the proximal nail fold. The groove continues to move distally as time goes on and the nail grows out. There is no specific treatment other than that of the underlying illness. Once the stressor is reduced, the Beau's groove will eventually grow out to the distal aspect of the nail and be removed with trimming of the free nail edge.

Splinter Hemorrhages—These small, thin, red, vertical lines can be $^1/_2$–4 mm long and initially appear at the proximal nail plate. Like Beau's grooves, they grow distally with the nail. Since these changes can be an embolic manifestation of bacterial endocarditis, this diagnosis should be ruled out. Splinter hemorrhages occur in otherwise healthy people as well. Thus, if endocarditis is not involved, one need not search further for another etiologic systemic illness. There exists no specific treatment.

Clubbing—Also known as Hippocratic fingers, these changes are usually seen in those patients with chronic lung disease. The free nail plate edge becomes somewhat curved, so it is rounded around the digit tip. Also, the area where the proximal nail plate joins the proximal nail fold becomes flattened. Finally, the digit itself becomes more wide and bulbous from the DIP joint distally. These changes are permanent and treating the underlying lung disease will not lead to any improvement.

Tumors—Various tumors can occur in the nail bed and they are quite common. Tumors in/around/under nails usually present with pain or throbbing. Often biopsy is necessary. This biopsy technique requires special skills/equipment and is probably most cost effective if performed by a dermatologist with a close relationship to those in dermatopathology. The most common is malignant melanoma. This malignancy, when involving the nail bed, presents as a black streak or nodule. Such black discoloration should be considered a melanoma until all other causes of black discoloration have been ruled out. Most other black discoloration is due to external staining of nail or dark foreign body under the nail. Treatment of tumors of the nail bed are best carried out by a dermatologist.

MANAGEMENT

To Manage

▼ Keep cases with defined etiology (other than tumor).

▼ Subungual Hematoma

Relieve pain via electrocautery.

Watch for secondary pyoderma.

▼ Oncolysis

Treat the underlying etiology (fungus, psoriasis, etc.).

▼ Paronychia

Fungal—Anticandidal antifungal (Lotrimin).

Apply 3 times daily for 2 weeks.

Do not bandage (open to air).

Bacterial—Twice daily, warm water soaks.

Oral antistaph antibiotics three times a day for 5–7 days.

I and D not necessary.

▼ Ingrown Toenail

1st visit: lift free edge, place cotton underneath.

Oral antistaph antibiotics 3 times daily for 5–7 days.

Soak twice daily in warm water.

2nd visit: surgical removal distal, lateral nail with Beaver Blade or surgical removal entire lateral nail plate.

Recheck in 1 week.

Patient education on toenail care for prevention.

▼ Herpetic Whitlow

Spontaneously resolve in 7–10 days.

Cool water/Burrow's solution soaks.

Oral analgesics PRN.

▼ Onychomycoses

Lamisil (Terbenafine) 150 mg orally a day for up to 12 weeks.

KOH to confirm prior to initiating therapy.

▼ Psoriasis

Treat skin lesions and nail changes usually resolve.

Injected steroid into nail fold helpful but possible pain and atrophy.

▼ Periungual Warts

Treat warts with cryotherapy or DNCB.

If long standing, nail deformity may not resolve.

▼ Beau's Grooves

No specific therapy.

Will grow out in 3–4 months.

▼ Splinter Hemorrhages

No specific therapy.

Will grow out in 3–4 months.

▼ Clubbing

No specific therapy.

Chronic, permanent change.

Send

▼ All suspected tumors for diagnosis and treatment

▼ Patients with psoriasis that requires UVB phototherapy, methotrexate, or PUVA

▼ If underlying etiology is questionable

PROGNOSIS

Depends on the etiology of the specific nail change. The above text included this information under sections II and III.

PEARLS AND PITFALLS

▼ KOH all changes associated with subungual increased keratin to rule out onychomycosis.

▼ The location of a Beau's groove can give insight into the time of its etiologic physiologic stressor.

▼ Although expensive, Lamisil is the premiere treatment for onychomycosis

▼ Although not necessary, electrocautery of subungual hematomas may relieve painful pressure.

CASE 6.6

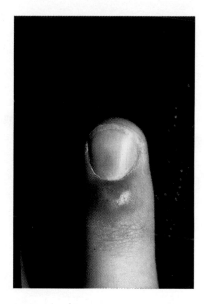

S: A 48-year-old female dental hygienist presents to your clinic with painful skin changes on her distal index finger. The rash developed about 3 days prior and she has never had a similar skin rash in the past. She denies any recent trauma to the affected digit. She has been placing topical antibiotic ointment on the rash at least 3 times each day. She is otherwise feeling well and has no other complaints. She feels a tender lump in her elbow.

O: The rash involves the periungual skin of the distal left index finger and consists of small (1–2mm diameter) vesicles. The underlying skin is red, warm, and swollen. The entire area is very tender to the touch. The rest of the skin is noted to be WNL. There is no axillary lymphadenopathy but some in the popliteal group. The rest of the exam is unremarkable as well.

A: Herpetic Whitlow

P: Cool water soaks every 4–6 hours.

Analgesia with 1000mg of oral Tylenol every 4–6 hours.

Reassurance that the lesion will spontaneously resolve in about 1 week.

May continue the topical antibiotic to prevent secondary pyoderma.

Consider antiherpes antibiotics if Whitlow recurs.

PATIENT EDUCATION HANDOUT
NAIL CHANGES

There exist many causes of nail changes—yours is due to/called _____.

Take all medication as instructed.

If you have a fungal infection, treatment is expensive. There is no risk to your health if you leave nail alone—the fungus will not spread and is not contagious. Treatment is up to you for cosmetic purposes only.

If you suffer from an ingrown toenail, proper toenail care is important

▼ Trim toenails regularly
▼ Do not trim closely—leave 3–5 mm of nail at the end of your toe
▼ Cut straight across
▼ After shower/bath, work out the end edges so they do not bend into your skin (ask your doctor how to do this).
▼ Wear shoes with proper width—avoid small, narrow toe box.

If you have a paronychia, do not try to pick or drain it on your own. Your doctor will do this if necessary. Take all of your medication until gone.

Call your doctor with *any* questions.

▶ PIGMENTARY PROBLEMS

Pigmentary abnormalities include both hyperpigmentation and hypopigmentation. The most common pigmentation skin abnormalities in the clinic are *chloasma, vitiligo,* and *pityriasis alba.* These will be discussed in the following chapter. There also exists hypo and hyperpigmentations, which are displayed as a part of complex genodermatoses or nevi. These are most often present from birth or later childhood. An example is the cafe-au-lait seen in neurofibromatosis. These pigmentary disorders are uncommonly seen in the primary care clinic and not included in the scope of this text.

▶ VITILIGO

BACKGROUND

Although this chronic hypopigmentary disease can affect the skin of all races, it appears to be more prevalent clinically in dark skinned individuals due to its cosmetic appearance. It can present as a cosmetic and social calamity for African Americans and it is important that the physician appreciates the comparable disfigurement. It can occur at any age and has no sexual predication, but often is familial. Some feel the vitiligo may have an autoimmune component, but this has not been proven. The most probable immune process mechanism would be the destruction of melanocytes. The Koebner phenomena has been seen in vitiligo patients, where the depigmentation occurs in areas of the skin after trauma.

IN THE CLINIC

Lesions typically present as white, round-to-segmented macules which may be as small as 1 mm in diameter and as large as to cover the entire sections of the body. There exists no overlying scale and vitiligo is asymptomatic. The lesions may occur anywhere on the body, but usually begin on the scrotum, vulva, finger-tips, and the backs of the hands. Often, lesion distribution is nearly symmetrical.

Patients may develop eye abnormalities, including iritis and chorioretinitis, and a few have subsequent hearing disorders. Any patient with ocular symptomology should be referred to an ophthalmologist to rule out such conditions. Also, many individuals with vitiligo have concurrent thyroid disease or auditory disorders. A thorough history, physical, and lab work-up should include consideration of possible thyroid abnormalities.

DIAGNOSIS AND TREATMENT

Vitiligo is almost always a clinical diagnosis. A differential for this skin hypopigmentation would most commonly include tinea versicolor, pityriasis alba, and chemical leukoderma. Tinea versicolor is usually pruritic and will have a positive KOH. Pityriasis alba rarely shows the complete white depigmentation seen in vitiligo. Finally, a patient with chemical leukoderma will give a history consistent with chemical exposure.

If the diagnosis is in question, skin biopsy is the diagnostic testing method. The biopsy demonstrated the total lack of melanocytes typical of vitiligo.

Treatment of vitiligo consists solely of PUVA therapy, either with oral or topical sensitizers. Thus, all patients with this skin disease are best referred to a dermatologist for their specialized, often costly and prolonged therapy. The primary care physician should conduct a thorough evaluation to rule out concurrent diseases such as thyroid abnormalities, anemia, and Addison's disease.

MANAGEMENT

▼ Keep—no patients who request cosmetic improvement. Plan for these requests.

▼ Perform thorough work up for thyroid disease, anemia, and Addison's disease as needed

Send

▼ All patients who desire cosmetic improvement

▼ Any patient with ocular complaints to an ophthalmologist

PROGNOSIS

Although one third of patients have *some* spontaneous repigmentation, most patients have chronic skin changes. The size and number of lesions may remain the same or increase. Unfortunately, the disease is unpredictable.

PEARLS AND PITFALLS

▼ A KOH is a simple, quick method to rule out tinea ersicolor.

▼ Any patient who desires cosmetic improvement requires PUVA and is best managed by a dermatologist.

▼ Consider cosmetic cover ups.

▶ PITYRIASIS ALBA

BACKGROUND

Pityriasis alba is a chronic skin disorder. It is a variant of mild eczema, which causes hypopigmentation. The disease is characterized by seasonal periods of exacerbation and remission. It develops as a result of the skin's reaction to inflammation. Pityriasis alba is seen mostly in children and some young adults and is often seen in those with atopic dermatitis. A mild eczema recurs on the face and lateral arms of these individuals and leads to the classic patchy depigmentation. Also, seborrheic dermatitis can produce P. alba in African American children.

IN THE CLINIC

The disease demonstrates small, patchy areas with partial loss of pigmentation. The macular lesions are poorly marginates and vary in size, number, and distribution. About $1/2$ the pigment is retained in patients with P. alba, while all is lost in those individuals with vitiligo (stark white). Scale is rarely present, but if involved is quite mild. Summer months show exacerbations. This apparent increase is due to the inability of these spots to tan. Thus, it is not an actual worsening of hypopigmentation. Rather, the areas with less pigment stand out against the tanned skin that surrounds them.

DIAGNOSIS AND TREATMENT

The diagnosis of P. alba is usually a clinical one. The lesions do mimic T. Versicolor and often parents express their concern over a possible "fungal" etiology. A KOH is usually warranted to rule out Tinea. Do not treat hypopigmented macules with an antifungal. If the loss of pigment is secondary to P. alba, topical antifungal preparations will worsen the disease and increase parental anxiety. Vitiligo involves macular hypopigmentation as well, but the affected spots are usually stark white, unlike the partial depigmentation of P. alba.

Treatment of pityriasis alba is the same as atopic dermatitis. Frequent, thorough use of lubricants and once to twice daily topical, mid-potency steroids are beneficial in resolving the scale and progression of the disease. But, there exists no treatment for the pigment loss. Any hypopigmentation that has occurred is chronic. There exists no reason to refer these patients unless the diagnosis is in question.

MANAGEMENT

- ▼ Keep all cases
- ▼ Treat with frequent lubrication
- ▼ Eliminate irritants (face scrubbing)
- ▼ Topical mid-potency steroids once to twice a day
- ▼ No treatment for hypopigmentation
- ▼ Rule out Tinea Versicolor with KOH exam

Send

Only for confirmation of diagnosis.

PROGNOSIS

Eczematous changes have an excellent prognosis with proper therapy as outlined above. The hypopigmentation is chronic and there currently exists no treatment to return the skin back to its normal color.

 CHLOASMA

BACKGROUND

Also known as melasma, this hyperpigmentary skin disorder occurs mainly in females (> 90% of cases) and has an increased frequency in brown skinned patients. Most patients are 18–35 years of age, though melasma can occur at any age. It is typically seen mostly in those patients who are pregnant or use oral contraceptives. Also, chloasma is seen more frequently in areas of the world with increased sun exposure and outdoor lifestyles. Some studies have shown diphenylhydantoin to be a precipitating factor as well.

Some individuals postulate a hormonal etiology for the skin changes of melasma. But, to date, no formal study has shown a specific mechanism between female hormones and the hyperpigmentation. Since oral contraceptives lead to melasma, it seems there is a hormonal reason behind the changes, but precise answers are not yet available. A familial tendency is seen.

IN THE CLINIC

The skin changes seen are a reticular hyperpigmentation consisting of brown to black, well defined macules. The lesions occur mainly on the face. The distribution is symmetrical and may be "mask-like" with involvement of the skin overlying the forehead, cheeks, upper lip, nose, and mandible. The skin changes are benign and have no malignant potential.

DIAGNOSIS AND TREATMENT

Diagnosis is almost always clinical. A careful history and examination will usually rule out other possible diagnoses for the hyperpigmentation. A Wood's lamp can be used to define the extent of the skin changes. Biopsy is diagnostic, but rarely necessary. Skin biopsy of melasma will demonstrate an increased number of melanocytes.

Treatment of chloasma can be done without specialist involvement. Many cases will spontaneously resolve over a period of months following delivery or discontinuation of hormone therapy. Treatment consists of Retin-A cream at a strength of .025% used at bedtime in combination with concomitant use of an opaque sunscreen whenever exposed to sunlight. One difficult issue is that any re-exposure of treated skin to sunlight without the use of an opaque sunscreen will lead to recurrence of the hyperpigmentation. Thus, even diseased skin faded with Retin-A therapy is susceptible to developing the same hyperpigmentation if exposed to sunlight without a sunscreen.

It is important to educate your patients so they have realistic treatment expectations. Make up used to conceal the hyperpigmentation is a reasonable option. Chemical facial peels have been used to correct chloasma. Although effective, again, the treated skin will re-develop the hyperpigmentation if exposed to the sun without sunscreen. Also, this option is quite expensive. Again, there exists no benefit in referral to a dermatologist.

MANAGEMENT

▼ Keep all cases
▼ Retin-A .025% qhs with use of opaque sunscreen whenever exposed to sunlight.
▼ Chemical peels
▼ Many cases spontaneously fade after delivery or discontinuance of oral contraceptive use.
▼ Must use opaque sunscreen religiously after Retin-A or chemical peel treatment to prevent recurrence.
▼ Referral not necessary

PROGNOSIS

As mentioned previously, many cases will spontaneously resolve when oral contraceptives are withdrawn or the pregnancy is over. Retin-A and chemical peel treatment is effective, but hyperpigmentation will recur if exposed to sunlight without an opaque sunscreen.

PEARLS AND PITFALLS

▼ Patient education is important for realistic treatment expectations.
▼ Any sunlight exposure without sunscreen after treatment will cause recurrence of hyperpigmentation. Sun avoidance is critical to any improvement.

CASE 6.7

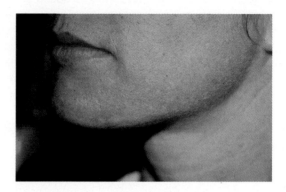

S: A 19-year-old female presents to your clinic in Savannah, Georgia in some emotional stress. She is extremely concerned over a number of dark spots that have been developing on her cheeks and upper lip. She states that the spots have been getting darker and darker over the past 2 months since she first noticed them. She is worried because the Magnolia Queen Beauty Contest is to be held in less than 1 month. She has been planning to enter the contest since she was a child and win just like her mother did when she was 18 years old. She has been attempting to cover the spots with make-up but it is not very effective. She states the skin changes are otherwise not bothersome in any manner and she has no other complaints. She does admit to frequenting a tanning bed at least 2 times each week to keep her "healthy glow" fresh for the competition. She has no medical illnesses and is on no medication except oral contraceptives which she began taking approximately 4 months prior to today's visit.

O: A pleasant, attractive blond female with significantly suntanned skin of entire body. No evidence of sunburn. The skin on her face displays dark brown macules ranging from 2–5 mm in diameter distributed symmetrically over her cheeks and upper lip. The spots are well circumscribed from the surrounding unaffected skin. The skin rash has no associated evidence of secondary change. The rest of the skin is WNL.

A: Chloasma

P: Advise stopping the oral contraceptive medication due to its causative association with this skin disease. Discuss other methods of birth control with the patient. Since the pageant is only 1 month away discuss the options with the patient. A chemical peel would leave her facial skin a significantly lighter shade than the skin over the rest of her body. Retin A cream is an option but the results obtained may not be significant enough by the time of the event. Either of these treatments will require her to remain out of the sun if the results are to be effective. Using make-up to hide the changes in addition is a viable option. Patient education on the evils of tanning and tanning beds in particular is important for this young woman.

PATIENT EDUCATION HANDOUT
PIGMENTARY PROBLEMS

The color change in your skin is due to a disease called:

_____

This skin disease is treated with the below therapies:

_____
_____
_____
_____

▶ PRURITUS

BACKGROUND

Pruritus is not itself a disease process rather it is a symptom of a disease. This sensation is commonly known as "itch" and can occur in any sex, gender, age group, or socio-economic class. Pruritus may occur along with a variety of skin diseases and often varies in its intensity from person to person. But, some patients who have absolutely no cutaneous changes can complain of pruritus as well. This phenomena is due to the fact that pruritus is a symptom of many systemic diseases that possess no clinical skin manifestation.

The clinical picture of pruritus is further confused by the fact that an itch will usually lead a patient to scratch their skin. Scratching an itchy area of skin will itself cause cutaneous changes. These cutaneous changes include irritation of nerve endings which stimulate more pruritus and more scratching. Thus, itch leads to scratch which leads to itch, and the itch-scratch cycle ensues. Via this itch-scratch cycle a patient who originally had no manifestations of rash can develop a non-specific lichenified eczema from their scratching of normal skin. On the same note, an individual who had initially developed a disease-specific pruritic rash can cause their typical manifestations to be blurred by their own secondary scratching response. Thus, a skin disease that was diagnostic in presentation may easily become difficult to diagnose if associated pruritus is severe enough to lead to secondary changes. Thus, we must approach pruritus in a systematic manner. Pruritus is best defined as organic or essential. It may also be further described as generalized or focal.

Organic Pruritus

Organic pruritus is itching that is associated with skin changes. The cutaneous manifestations of a certain skin disease may be apparent at the onset of the pruritus as in (tinea pedis, scabies, pityriasis rosea, or chigger bites), or the pruritus may occur a period of time after the itching begins (anaphylaxis, pemphigoid, drug eruptions, lymphoma, phototoxicity).

Essential Pruritus

This subtype of pruritus is the itch that occurs although there is no apparent associated dermatitis. This is "pure itch." The classic example is xerosis, or dry skin. Xerosis is common in the aged population, especially in the winter months. This group of patients have skin that heals poorly and is less prone to hidrosis. Also, the elderly are often bored and or depressed which can lead to an increased fixation on subsequent scratching behavior. Xerosis is more severe in the winter months due to the low humidity of heated environments with further decrease in overall skin hidrosis. An elderly individual may actually present at an advanced stage of xerosis that can be classified as a form subclinical irritant eczema known commonly as "senile pruritus with eczema."

Essential pruritus is usually generalized as listed in Table 6.1. Other important causes of essential pruritus include metabolic/endocrine factors, neoplasms, infestations, drugs, hepatic diseases, hematologic diseases, pregnancy related disorders, and psychogenic disorders.

Generalized Pruritus

When the itch is present over the entire body surface rather than one single area, it is generalized.

Focal Pruritus

When the itch is restricted to a fixed, focal area of skin, it is focal pruritus. For example a spot on the back, pruritus ani, or itchy nipples, nape of the neck, or soles of feet.

IN THE CLINIC

When the skin rash is examined it usually consists of one of two basic lesions—eczema or urticaria. Refer to the introduction for a review of these topics.

DIAGNOSIS AND TREATMENT

Proper diagnosis of pruritus begins with a thorough history taking effort on the part of the physician. It is quite important to determine if the patient began experiencing the itching before the rash, after the rash, or without any skin changes whatsoever. Look carefully at all the skin. The etiology of most organic pruritus is usually determined without significant effort. The cause of an essential prutitus is often much more difficult to delineate. Ask about other symptoms over the recent months including fatigue, fever, malaise, mood changes, ab-

TABLE 6.1 ▼ Differential Diagnosis of Essential Pruritis

Malignancies
  Lymphomas (Hodgkin and non-Hodgkin varieties)
  Leukemia
  Mastocytosis multiple myelinoma
  GI, CNS, lung tumors
Metabolic disease
  Thyroid (hypo. or hyper)
  Hyperparathyroidism
  Diabetes mellitus
Infestations
  Scabies
  Hookworm
  Ascaris
  Lice
Drugs (subclinical sensitivity)
  Alcohol
  Morphine
  Codeine
  Thiamine, niacin in large doses
  Scopolamic
Hepatic disease
  Any subclinical jaundice
Chronic renal failure
Hematologic
  Polycythemia vera
  HIV (multiple)
  Anemia—iron deficiency
Psychogenic
  Delusions of parasitosis
  Neurotic excoriation
  Stress
Pregnancy
  PUPPP early
  Pre-prurigo of pregnancy
  Cholecystosis of pregnancy

dominal pain, headache, or weight loss. Also review medication list for any possible suspect drugs.

After a thorough history is taken a pertinent physical examination and close skin survey should be performed. A brief generalized over-look in addition to a close examination of the skin changes is adequate in most cases of organic pruritus. As with the history taking above, a physician must perform much more thorough physical examination in cases of essential pruritus. Essential pruritus will often require laboratory investigation as well as which labs to perform (CBC, LFTs, RFTs, thyroid screens, serum glucose, etc.) will depend on the findings of the history and physical examination.

The diagnosis of generalized essential pruritus may be quite elusive. The patient afflicted with this symptom is often in significant distress. The severity of the itch can be so intense it may lead to insomnia, anxiety, and depression. Be aware and sensitive to these issues in the patient with this wholly involving and quite debilitating symptomatology.

Often an area of fixed, organic pruritus can be approached diagnostically based on where the exact patch of skin is located. The most common of these organic pruritus and their most probable diagnosis follow:

Area of pruritus	Probable diagnosis	Treatment
Ear canals	Seborrheic dermatitis	pg ____
Nape of neck	Folliculitis	pg ____
Soles of feet/ toe webs	Tinea pedis	pg ____
Waistline	Irritant contact dermatitis	pg ____
Nipples	Irritant contact dermatitis	pg ____
Vulva/penis	STD/psychogenic/ intertrigo	pg ____
Anus (pruritus ani)	Irritant dermatitis C.D. (Stool soiling)	pg ____

Specific treatment of pruritus is dependent on the exact diagnosis. The etiology of the itch must first be determined via the aforementioned methods. Then, the specific cause is approached in a tailored manner. Please refer to specific chapters themselves for the diagnosis-based treatment protocols. If xerosis is determined to be the etiology the patient is best approached as if they were experiencing atopic dermatitis (i.e., lubricate, lubricate, lubricate), and judge the result.

The pruritus can be treated as well. Most patients are more concerned with the acute resolution of the itching than the determination of its cause. As with xerosis, frequent lubrication with a cream or ointment is very helpful. Topical mid potency steroid creams liberally applied twice each day are often necessary. Oral antihistamines are almost always recommended. Unfortunately the sedating forms are significantly more palliative then the non-sedating varieties. Often a sedating antihistamine aids with the insomnia experienced by the pruritic patient. The recent empiric use of H^2 antagonists to reduce pruritus has no sound evidence base and is not helpful. Prepare to spend a long time in assuring and helping the practice patient to implement care.

MANAGEMENT

To Manage

▼ Keep all
1. Focal, organic causes
2. Generalized organic causes
3. Essential causes responsive to therapy in 2–3 weeks

▼ Treatment
1. Determine underlying rash/systemic illness. Aim for "disease-specific" treatment.
2. In general—reduce pruritus

    Lubricate, Lubricate, Lubricate

    Topical mid-potency corticosteroids BID

    Oral H_1 antihistamines every 8 hours as needed (drowsy formulas may help with insomnia)

Send

▼ Any essential pruritus that cannot be controlled at all via above methods.
▼ Any essential pruritus non-responsive after 2–3 weeks of appropriate treatment.
▼ Any essential pruritus not diagnosed within 2 office visits for consultation.

PROGNOSIS

Unfortunate if the prognosis is dependent on the available treatment of the underlying skin rash/systemic disease. Pruritus can become chronic and debilitating—causing both patient and physician frustration.

If the itching is localized and the patient scratches frequently and vigorously, *neurodermatitis* may develop. Neurodermatitis refers to the formation of chronic, lichenified plaques as a sequela to local trauma caused by the scratching. If the scratching is stopped, the neurodermatitis will resolve. The majority of neurodermatitis is secondary and common causes include atopic dermatitis, folliculitis, and allergic contact dermatitis. Neurodermatitis can be primary as well. Although rare, the etiology of primary neurodermatitis is psychogenic. These patients develop the typical chronic skin changes as a result of repetitive scratching of wholly normal skin and lack of any underlying systemic disease or other pathological factor. This diagnosis is always one of exclusion. Psychotherapy is disappointing.

CASE 6.8

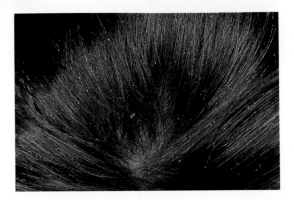

S: A 4-year-old female presents to your clinic with her mother. She has been complaining of an itchy scalp for about a week. The itch has been getting worse and the mother is concerned because her daughters skin around her neck and hyalin is becoming more and more red. The patient admits to scratching frequently. Her mother treated her with an over the counter product for lice about 10 days prior due to an outbreak at the day care.

O: Well nourished, pleasant young female. Afebrile. Skin, scalp, and posterior neck demonstrates diffuse erythematous patches with poor margination and moderate excoriation. No lymphallenopathy. Hair shafts with nits/lice present. Exam is otherwise WNL.

A: Lice with secondary irritant dermatitis

P: Treat lice with product of your choice. Atarax every 8 hours until skin changes improve.

▼
PATIENT EDUCATION HANDOUT
PRURITUS

The itch you are having is due to _____.

It is important to take all medications as your doctor has instructed.

Other information that is helpful:

▶ ROSACEA

BACKGROUND

Rosacea is the result of a functional vascular anomaly in the central face with a strong predisposition to involve the follicles and their stroma. Gradually, a chronic acneform rash develops. Lesions cluster on the chin, forehead, ears, and most typically in the "butterfly" pattern of the face. In regards to bacteriology, lipid content, and histopathology, rosacea is similar to adolescent acne. It is more common in females and patients are usually 25 years or older. It tends to have a familial predisposition and is more common in pale skinned people. African Americans have a reduced incidence of rosacea, so some postulate that long time sun damage may be an etiology. Endocrine factors may be another. We notice a greater prevalence of A. pylori infections in rosacea patients, and this may be clinically important in managing patients unresponsive to routine treatments. Gastric disturbances are common with rosacea. Improving digestion may help the rosacea.

About 50% of patients with rosacea also have chronic periodic facial flushing with various oral stimuli. Thus, diet is important in these people. Patients need to avoid hot or ice drinks, alcohol, coffee, tea, strong spices, and seafood. For other patients, sunburn, chilling and windburn are predisposing factors and should be minimized. Rosacea is often seasonal, mainly in summertime.

Gradually, the chronic inflammation will cause fibrosis which accumulates over the years to form rhinophyma. Rhinophyma or "potato nose" is much more common in males than in females. People with rosacea may also notice irritation of the eyes, inflammation of eyelids, and visual disturbances. The reason for such eye involvement is currently not known, but may be due to irritant keratitis. Usually, eye signs occur only in those patients with longstanding disease.

IN THE CLINIC

Lesions of rosacea include a generalized macular erythema with superimposed erythematous papules, nodules and telangiectasias. Pustules are rare, and if present, are tiny and form the top of a papule. There are no comedones present. The lesions are discrete and found in a typical "butterfly" pattern with symmetrical involvement of the cheeks, nose, ears, brows, and chin. Men can develop rhino-phyma, which was discussed above.

Lesions may last days to weeks and continue to form in a chronic nature if left untreated. Treatment will improve the lesions, but if discontinued, the rosacea almost always reappears eventually.

DIAGNOSIS AND TREATMENT

Two differential diagnostic considerations are infection (erysipelas) and lupus erythematosus. Erysipelas is intensively painful, crusted, and causes severe eyelid edema and lymphadenopathy, as a rule. Also, erysipelas is seldom symmetrical or patterned (forehead and chin spot). Lupus is seldom pustular, but is scarring and atrophic, as well as scaling. Look in ears and over scalp for other lesions of lupus. Rosacea patients often have some mild incidental arthritis, and older patients may have marginal ANA tests. Rosacea is evanescent and loaded with sensations of heat and flushing, while lupus is not. Usually the diagnosis is clear, but biopsy is the decisive procedure to decide about lupus. Facial tinea and allergy to cosmetics may mimic rosacea occasionally.

The first line of treatment for rosacea is oral tetracycline at doses of 500–1000 mg per day. Unfortunately, many older patients do not tolerate this highly effective antibiotic. Amoxicillin at similar doses may be substituted. These oral antibiotics help decrease the papules and papulopustules of rosacea. The response to oral therapy is quicker than in juvenile acne with 2—3 weeks of treatment demonstrating notable improvement.

The underlying redness and telengestasias are treated with topical metridnidazole gel or cream (0.75%) applied one or two times daily. This topical preparation is quite effective. Often, once the papules, pustules, and nodules have resolved on oral antibiotics, a patient can be maintained on this topical preparation only. But, if a patient has a significant recurrence, oral antibiotics must be restarted.

If rosacea is severe, the patient should be referred to a dermatologist for possible Accutane therapy. If a female patient with rosacea suffers from a significant predisposition to flushing episodes, the addition of estrogen may aid in the overall treatment regimen. Men with rhinophyma have the option of cosmetic surgery after the disease is well controlled.

MANAGEMENT

▼ Keep all cases without severe involvement or ophthalmological symptoms.

▼ Initiate oral antibiotics:

1st line—tetracycline 500–1000 mg a day

Amoxicillin 500–1000 mg a day if cannot tolerate tetracycline

▼ Start topical metridnidazole .075% gel or cream, apply one to two times daily.

▼ Consider estrogen replacement for women with excessive flushing symptoms.

Send

▼ Severe cases without improvement in 8 weeks

▼ Rhinophyma for cosmetic surgery

▼ If a granulomatous component, eye involvement to ophthalmologist

PROGNOSIS

Very good if patient is compliant. Long term topical therapy after initial improvement in combination with oral antibiotics should be expected. If outbreak occurs, restart oral antibiotics until well controlled. Rhinophyma requires cosmetic surgery as previously outlined.

PEARLS AND PITFALLS

▼ Always start with oral antibiotics in conjunction with topical metridnidazole for best result

▼ Never use tetracycline, metronidazole or accutane in pregnant patients.

▼ If de-pigmentation is severe, reconsider the possibility of lupus.

▼ Re-consider the coexistence of ulcerative disease of the stomach when rosacea recurs.

▼ Ask again about eyesight at each visit.

▼ If scaling is heavy, always do the KOH examination.

CASE 6.9

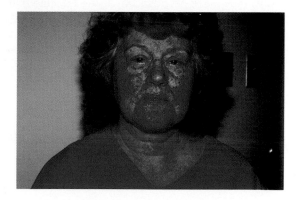

S: A 33-year-old female fisherman patient presents to your clinic in Bar Harbor, Maine with complaints of "acne." She states that she never had problems with acne as a teenager but began noticing acne like skin changes about 6 months prior. She has tried numerous OTC acne medications but they all seem to just dry out her skin. She is part-owner of a small fleet of fishing boats and is often required to man a haul when an employee is absent. She does state that the rash is the worst on those days that follow such shifts on the boat. Also, she admits that the rash seems worse after she has been eating fresh seafood or drinking a beer with her shipmates. She is otherwise healthy and takes no medication on a regular basis.

O: A pleasant female who appears older than her stated age. The patients skin over her face shows numerous erythematous papules distributed within a macular erythema on the skin of the nose, paranasal area, chin, and forehead in a somewhat symmetrical fashion. There is one 5mm diameter nodule on the left chin that is nonmobile and is not tender to palpation. She has a 3mm diameter telangiectasia on her right cheek. You find no pustules or comedonal lesions. Other than numerous scars on her hands from working the nets and cleaning/sorting the catch the rest of her skin is WNL.

A: Rosacea.

P: Start oral antibiotics—Tetracycline 500mg twice each day. Warn about sunscreens. Start topical metronidazole cream .075% twice each day. Advise avoiding the wind and sun whenever possible or at least employing a hat and a sunscreen liberally when working in such conditions. Also, advise that seafood, spices, hot/cold beverages, and alcohol may make her rosacea worse. Educate that results are not always seen until 4 to 6 weeks of treatment. Patient to follow up for recheck in 6 weeks.

PATIENT EDUCATION HANDOUT
ROSACEA

The skin changes you have are a form of adult type acne known as Rosacea.

This skin disease requires treatment long-term. If you stop using your medicine the rash will eventually return.

Your doctor has prescribed a gel/cream called metronidazole for your skin. You should apply this medication:

Twice a day
Once a day

Your doctor has prescribed an oral antibiotic called

_____ .

This medication should be taken _____

_____ .

If you become pregnant stop the medication immediately and phone your physician

Make a follow-up appointment in _____ _____ .

Call if you have any questions or concerns.

▶ Viral Exanthems

BACKGROUND

This group of diseases are placed in a single chapter of this text due to their similar presentations and treatment. Here we will discuss these exanthems (cutaneous) and enanthems (mucocutaneous) that are caused by viral infections. Often the same virus may lead to different skin changes in different patients due to variations in immunity between separate individuals. Also, similar exanthems can be caused by viral, bacterial or metazoal infection, insect bites, allergic food/dry reactions, and autoimmune diseases. "Viral exanthem" is over diagnosed.

Thus, confusion over the etiology of a specific exanthem is probable. Physicians must not only look at the rash itself, but at other factors such as historical data, physical finding, exposure, and laboratory values to distinguish between a viral etiology and another possible causative agent. Once determined to be part of a viral syndrome, the exact virus is usually narrowed down based on some of the findings discussed in the following chapter. Necessary treatment of all viral exanthems is purely supportive. Rest, analgesics, antipyretics, antihistamines, and cool soaks are usually all that is required to treat viral exanthems until they spontaneously resolve.

It is important to carefully document in the patient's chart, the data of any exanthem and whether the patterns of rash and symptomatology will allow diagnosis of the specific etiology. Also, be certain to chart immunization status, even in your nonpediatric population.

The text that follows will cover those viral exanthems most commonly encountered in the primary care clinic. Unlike other chapters of this book, the background, clinical appearance, treatment and prognosis are all covered in a single section under each specific viral etiology. Varicella Zoster infection (chicken pox / shingles) has been discussed in a previous section and will only be mentioned briefly.

DIAGNOSIS AND TREATMENT

Epstein-Barr Virus (EBV)

This member of the Herpes virus family is typical in its almost universal presence in patients by adulthood. Approximately 50% of patients seroconvert by age 5 years. EBV is not highly contagious and it is thought that most spread occurs via intimate contact. Many infections are subclinical in nature and the affected individual is not ever seen in the office.

The most common clinical manifestation of EBV is as infectious mononucleosis. Known to many as "mono," this disease is usually seen in teenagers, but may present at any age. The classic clinical triad includes pharyngitis, lymphadenopathy, and fever. Another common complaint is severe fatigue. Other findings include headache, myalgias, and hepatosplenomegaly. It is worthwhile to examine the mouth because about 50% of patients develop palatial petechia. Only 10% actually show the skin changes of a febrile exanthem.

If a rash is present, it is usually widespread, begins on the face and neck, spreads to the trunk, and finally to the extremities. It will consist of erythematous, well demarcated papules with a slight macular nature. The rash is very faint and is not pruritic or painful. 90% of patients with EBV, when treated with ampicillin, will develop a widespread, significant rubelliform rash as a result of the antibiotic therapy.

The course of infectious mononucleosis is 1–3 weeks in length and most patients fully recover by then. The fatigue often persists longer. Complications rarely occur, but some patients may develop splenic rupture, airway obstruction, hepatic changes, and thrombocytopenia.

Measles

Unlike EBV, this viral syndrome is very contagious. It is due to infection with a paramyxovirus and spread to unaffected individuals via airborne droplets. Although immunization exists, many children and older teenagers have not been fully vaccinated and can contract the disease. Humans are the only reservoir of this viral disease.

Measles has two distinct clinical stages which follow the 10–12 day incubation period. Initially, a 2–4 day prodrome of fever, cough, photophobia, anorexia, malaise, coryza, conjunctivitis, and an enanthem occurs. The enanthem is known as Koplick's spots. These lesions are 2–3 mm diameter blue-grey papules on a typical erythematous base. The Koplick's spots are initially seen on the buccal mucosa and eventually spread throughout the entire oropharynx.

The second stage begins about 2 days after the Koplick's spots occur and consists of the typical erythematous macular skin changes.

These begin on the face and proceed down to the trunk and finally to the extremities. The macules can become more papular as they spread. The generalized rash lasts about 4–7 days and resolves in the same pattern as it occurs (ie. head downwards). The prodromal symptoms mentioned above continue and heighten when the rash is at its peak and will resolve at the same time the skin changes do.

Patients can appear extremely ill, and the fever can be quite high. Common complications include otitis media, pneumonia, and encephalitis. Myocelitis can occur but is rare. The disease is otherwise self-limited and resolves spontaneously. Treatment is supportive only, with pain control, hydration, and antipyretics. No specific antiviral agent exists.

Prophylaxis is recommended. A live measles vaccine should be administered at age 15 months and again when entering elementary school. Born after 1957, an individual should have received a measles vaccination after 1 year of age. Most colleges and universities require a second measles vaccine for those who received only 1 before entry.

Rubella (German Measles)

Like Rubeola, this viral infection is highly contagious and spread via airborne droplets. It occurs mostly in children and young adults, although outbreaks have been greatly reduced via available immunization. Unlike Rubeola, this viral syndrome is characterized by very mild systemic symptoms that are usually benign. In most cases, an infection is subclinical.

The incubation period for Rubella is 2–3 weeks. This time is followed by mild upper respirator symptoms, low fever, malaise, lymphadenopathy and painful lateral and upwards gaze. The prodrome lasts 2–3 days and is followed by a mild, generalized, lightly erythematous maculopapular rash. The skin changes begin on the face and then move to the trunk and finally the extremities. The rash lasts 2–3 days and fully resolves. Constitutional symptoms continue during the exanthem. An enanthem of soft palatal petechia can occur and is known as Forsheimer's sign.

The most significant complication is congenital rubella syndrome. A fetus is most at risk for developing this complication if its mother was exposed to the virus during the first trimester of pregnancy. The congenital rubella syndrome is characterized by low birth weight, hepatosplenomegaly, thrombocytopenia, mental retardation, deafness, seizures, cataracts, and behavioral disorders. Any pregnant female who is uncertain of her rubella status should have it checked during the initial physician visit. Treatment of the postnatal syndrome is supportive only. No anti-viral therapy exists. The live vaccine is administered at 15 months and again when entering grade school.

Erythema Infectiosum (Fifth Disease)

This familiar viral syndrome occurs as a result of infection with Parvovirus B-19. This virus can also lead to chronic hemolytic anemia, and acute arthropathy, and hydrops fetalis, but erythema infection is the most common manifestation of Parvovirus B-19.

Erythema infectiosum is usually self-limited and most commonly seen in children under the age of 12 years. It is spread via respiratory droplets and is moderately contagious in nature until the rash appears. An incubation period of about 14 days is followed by the sudden eruption of the exanthem. A prodromal phase of fever and malaise may occur, but is not always present.

The exanthem begins as an extremely bright red macular change of the skin on the cheeks and chin only. This gives the child the "slap-cheek" appearance that this disease is known for. The facial changes are followed by an erythematous maculopapular rash over the extremities (mostly extensor surfaces) and possibly the trunk. The central areas begin to fade over a few days and the typical "lacy" or "fern-leaf" pattern occurs. This change is seen most commonly on the extremities and not the trunk.

The entire exanthem clears in about a week, but may reappear transiently in the following 1–2 months without any constitutional hallmarks. Reassurance of the parents is the only necessity of treatment. Rarely are children ill enough that they need to be withheld from school or activity. As previously mentioned, hydrops fetalis can occur in a pregnant woman who is exposed to an individual who is infected. The pregnant patient should be tested. If serologically positive they will require close follow-up with further investigation to rule out this possible complication. Some patients have arthralgias, sustained fatigue and neurologic symptoms for some months.

Roseola Infantum

This viral syndrome is due to infection with human herpes virus 6 (HHV6) and 90% of patients are between 6 and 18 months of age. It is the most common viral exanthem seen in young children.

It has a significant febrile prodrome that may be accompanied by malaise and anorexia as well. The high fever precedes the rash by about 3 days. Usually, the patients constitutional symptoms are nearly resolved when the rash occurs. The exanthem consists of erythematous maculopapular changes that are limited to the upper trunk and neck. Unlike most of the other viral exanthems, roseola does not manifest or extremity skin changes. The rash is transient, lasting hours to a few days and is nonpruritic in nature.

Treatment of roseola is supportive only. The high fever has been known to induce febrile seizures, so antipyretics are necessary and important. Complications are rare and patients usually recover without further difficulties.

Varicella Zoster Virus (chicken pox)

This viral syndrome is caused by the herpes virus varicella zoster. It has been fully discussed in its own separate chapter 8.10. Please refer to the previous text for further details. It has been mentioned here due to its classification as a febrile exanthem.

Enterovirus

Enteroviruses that cause viral exanthems include echovirus, enterovirus, and Coxsackie virus. These agents are the most common cause of febrile exanthems in children in the summer and early fall. Such infections are extremely common and all are spread via the fecal-oral route.

These viral syndromes are clinically similar and it is rarely important to distinguish which inciting agent is responsible. They all last about 4–5 days and begin with the sudden onset of fever, diarrhea, nausea, emesis, mild abdominal pain, pharyngitis, myalgias and lymphadenopathy. The exanthem begins early and is characterized by spread from the face to the trunk and extremities. The actual appearance of the rash varies with the responsible infecting agent and can be rubelliform, macular or papular. Most of the exanthems are not distinctive enough to determine which enterovirus is responsible. Since the diseases are self-limited and treatment is similar in all cases, the determination of the exact agent responsible is rarely necessary.

Coxsackie A viruses are an exception to the above rule. These agents are responsible for "hand-foot-and-mouth" disease and herpangina. In herpangina a 2 day prodrome of sudden onset of fever and malaise is followed by a typical enanthem. Erythematous macules develop on the palate, buccal surfaces and tongue. The macules typically vesiculate and eventually erode and ulcerate. The lesions are extremely painful and patients have a hard time eating and drinking. Malaise may be impressive and long listing. Patients may become dehydrated, needing parenteral fluids.

In "hand-foot-and-mouth" disease, the enanthem above appears in concert with a typical exanthem. The rash is seen as small, round vesicles that are nonpruritic and usually displayed over the lateral aspects of the hands and feet. In herpangina, the above exanthem occurs in concert with a rubelliform rash that spreads from the face to the trunk and extremities. The exanthem is also nonpruritic. In both of these Coxsackie A infections, the rash resolves within about 1–1½ weeks.

All enteroviral infections have no specific therapy. Rather supportive care is indicated. Complications are very rare and most patients are back to normal within 2 weeks at the outset, or with herpangina in adults, perhaps 4 weeks.

PEARLS AND PITFALLS

▼ Drug eruptions closely mimic exanthems. If a patient is already ill and on an antibiotic, the best decision is to stop or change those drugs most likely to produce the rash. Reevaluated over 5 days time. There are no useful laboratory tests and biopsy is not helpful.

▼ Severe erythemas: Scalded skin syndrome from staphylococcal infections and toxic epidermal neurolysis (drugs) may resemble exanthems initially. Both develop into a bullous and exfoliative morphology.

▼ Showers of purpura:

About 90% of patients with meningococcemia show red spots on the skin, followed by showers of primary purpura.

Rocky Mountain Spotted Fever and other rickettsial illnesses have a widespread red-spotted macular rash that promptly becomes purpuric.

Gonococcemia classically produces a small pustule central to a patch of purpura. These skin changes are usually seen around large joints.

Subacute bacterial endocarditis will produce purpuric nodules and splinter hemorrhages due to emboli.

▼ A classic toxic generalized maculopapular eruption is often seen after insect or arthropod stings. This rash can resemble the effect of bacterial toxins or inflammatory skin reactions.

▼ Older people and children with chronic eczema are especially prone to allergic disseminations of the disease. This dissemination may resemble and exanthem. These flares are most common with nickel allergy, stasis dermatitis, and active atopic dermatitis. Very Acute contact dermatitis (poison ivy) can produce an exanthem-like rash, but usually the presence of pustules aids in the correct diagnosis. Less important mimics of exanthems include miliaria, multiple bug bites and exaggerated vasomotor reactions.

CASE 6.10

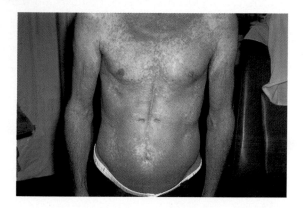

S: A 19-year-old freshman football player at Miami University (Ohio) presents again to the student health service complaining of a 10-day history of a "very-bad" sore throat, lumps in his neck, and exceptional fatigue. He even says it is difficult to swallow his high protein milk shakes. He aches all over, but he plays at defensive tackle, and always aches all over. Four days ago, at Student Health Service he received ampicillin for his sore throat. His girl friend, a freshman cheerleader, has become sick with the same severe fatigue. He has had no abdominal pain or dyspnea. He does state that he has felt hot, but has not taken his temperature. His girlfriend has been feeling tired over the last 2 days as well. He has been sleeping 10 hours and still is not rested. He missed practice the last 3 days and his coach is threatening to not let him start this Saturday if he misses any more. He asks you for "an antibiotic or something" to help.

O: Well nourished and muscular, but pale and diaphoretic. Feels warm: Temp—101.3 F orally. Shows no other abnormalities. Skin: Diffuse, widespread, symmetrical papulosquamous erythematous. Lesions all in one stage. Changes: Presence of excoriation and eyelid edema with tiny macular purpura on his palate.

HEENT—posterior oropharynx is erythematous and extremely edematous. There is no enanthem or tonsillar exudates. The rest of the HEENT is WNC. *neck*—#2—1 cm posterior cervical lymph nodes on the right and #3—$\frac{1}{2}$ cm posterior cervical lymph nodes on the left. FROM—supple
lungs—Clear, anterior and posterior
cu—RRR. No murmur. There is an S$_3$ gallop.
abd—soft, BS+ nontender. Well developed "6-pack" abdominal muscles

lead to difficulty in exam, but no apparent organomegaly. Spleen not palpable. A km lymph nodes are found in the neck, right axilla and the left inguinal regions; *ext*—warm, no edema, no cyanosis; *lab*—EBV titer—negative; CBC—WBC—18.3; H/H —WNC
gran—76.3%; lymph—18.1%; mono—6.2%; quick strep—negative; strep culture—negative.

A: Infectious Mononucleosis with amphicillin drug rash

P:

▼ Inform coach of diagnosis

▼ No class or practice for 1 week and review case.

▼ Recheck in 1 week

▼ Relative rest until recheck

▼ Tylenol or Ibuprofen as needed for fever and pain

▼ Push fluids

▼ Oral antihistamine every 8 hours for itch.

▼ Remember giving antibiotics to these patients predisposes to adverse cutaneous drug eruptions.

▼ Lozenges or salt water gargles for sore throat

▼ If any abdominal pain or symptoms worsen—call immediately.

NOTE: EBV titer often takes 14 days to show positive.

PATIENT EDUCATION HANDOUT
VIRAL EXANTHEMS

This name, viral exanthem, is the technical "doctor" term for an illness with a group of physical findings, one of which is a rash.

There are many types of viruses which can cause an "exanthem." Often we cannot determine *exactly* which virus is responsible.

Knowing the exact virus is not always important because the way to treat all of these is similar.

_____Your (child's) rash is probably caused by the specific virus _____ and is called _____. Write this down in the shot record.

_____Your (child's) rash is due to a virus whose exact name is not important to document.

Follow the treatment outlined by your physician. Call if any fever is above 101.5 degrees F and does not reduce with Tylenol or Ibuprofen.

An effective way to lower fever that is high or continues to return is to give a dose of Tylenol every 6 hours and a dose of Ibuprofen every 6 hours. *BUT* alternate the medication. So, you are getting 1 or the other every 3 hours.

For example:

    12:00—Tylenol
    3:00—Ibuprofen
    6:00—Tylenol
    9:00—Ibuprofen
    Etc.

Continue for 24 hours. Then use one or the other as needed only.

▶ ZOSTERS—HERPES AND VARICELLA

▶ HERPES ZOSTER

BACKGROUND

Herpes zoster is an acute infection caused by the same varicella zoster virus (VZV) which is responsible for chicken pox (varicella). While a patient has chicken pox, the varicella zoster virus moves from the epidermis to the dorsal nerve root of the sensory ganglia. The DNA virus will then lay dormant in the dorsal nerve root until reactivated. The latent varicella zoster virus, when reactivated, will travel back down the sensory nerves to the skin from which it originally rose. The typical dermatomal pain and vesiculobullous eruption of herpes zoster results.

Most patients will be 40 years of age or older and there is no sexual or racial predilection. Herpes zoster may appear without a possible reason for reactivation of the virus. Usually, a predisposing factor exists. Such predisposition includes immunosuppression (especially HIV patients), psychological/physical stress, trauma to sensory ganglia, and old age.

As with varicella zoster, herpes zoster is contagious. An individual exposed to herpes zoster who has never had varicella infection in the past may become infected and contract varicella. These individuals will display varicella, not a primary herpes zoster infection. They may develop zoster later in life due to the same mechanism as a primary varicella infection. Contact with an individual who has a herpes zoster outbreak will not lead to "primary" herpes zoster in the exposed individual. Nor will it lead to another varicella infection in a person who has had varicella zoster in the past.

IN THE CLINIC

The most common symptoms include sudden pain, paraesthesia, and a pruritic rash. Headache, fever, and fatigue may also occur. The pain and paraesthesia usually will begin 2–5 days before the rash is visualized.

The pain can be both severe and debilitating. The rash itself is unilateral and dermatomal. The herpetic lesions occur on an erythematous, edematous base. They start out as tender, red papules which change quickly into clustered umbilicated vesicles and eventually to pustules. The pustules break down in 7–10 days after which crusts weeping are displayed. Regional lymph nodes can be enlarged as well.

As noted above, herpes zoster is dermatomal. Although the T_6 thoracic nerve root is the most commonly affected dermatome, the ophthalmic branch of the trigeminal nerve is the most dangerous. Herpes zoster infection of this cranial nerve root can lead to severe ophthalmological complications, such as corneal ulcers, keratitis, conjunctivitis, scleritis, or iridocyclitis. These patients should be immediately referred to the ophthalmologist. Other dangerous nerve root involvement includes those of the genitals and the palms or soles.

If herpes zoster occurs during the first trimester of pregnancy, the fetus is at risk for secondary developmental anomalies. This topic should be discussed at length with any pregnant women who develop a herpes zoster breakout at this point in their pregnancy. If these women are promptly treated with oral antiviral agents, the likelihood of fetal anomalies is reduced, but full data is lacking. The possible development of post herpetic neuralgia will be discussed in the prognosis (V) section of this chapter.

DIAGNOSIS AND TREATMENT

The typical prodrome of pain can be confusing, especially in patients experiencing herpes zoster for the first time. The pain has been wrongfully diagnosed as pulmonary, cardiac, and musculoskeletal disease, to name a few.

The herpes zoster rash is similar to that caused by a herpes simplex virus infection. Location and the associated prodromal symptoms of herpes zoster may aid in distinguishing the tow viral rashes. Although Tzanck smears are positive in both herpes zoster and simplex, viral cultures will be diagnostic. VZV is very difficult to culture, while HSV is easily cultured.

Treatment of herpes zoster is mainly symptomatic. Cool water or Burow's solution soaks 3 times daily, oral analgesics, and oral antihistamines are usually sufficient therapeutic measures. Although the infection spontaneously resolves, the initiation of oral antivirals within 96 hours of symptom onset is essential in reducing the severity and time course of the disease. Oral Valacyclovir should be given at doses of 1.0 g (2 tabs.), 3 times daily, for 7 days. Oral Acyclovir has been shown to be less effective than Valcyclovir in treating herpes zoster infections. All patients should be educated about the possible recurrence of the disease, its predisposing factors and the possible complications that are discussed in section V of this chapter.

MANAGEMENT

To Manage

▾ Keep all cases without ophthalmic involvement and if nondisseminated

▾ Symptomatic treatment

▾ Cool water or Burow's solution soaks TID

▾ Moderate analgesia

▾ Oral antihistamines

▾ Try to treat patients at *earliest* possible time

▾ If within 96 hours of symptoms

  Oral valcyclovir 500 mg 2 tabs TID three times daily for 7 days

  Acyclovir not as effective as Valcyclovir

▾ Patient Education

  May recur, but uncommon

  Notify physician during prodrome if possible to initiate oral antivirals early.

  In all pregnant patients, inform about risk of fetal anomalies if first trimester infection

Send

▾ Eye involvement to ophthalmologist (urgent)

▾ Disseminated or necrotic cases to dermatologist

PROGNOSIS

The lesions of herpes zoster and the associated pain, paraesthesia, and pruritus usually spontaneously resolve in 7 days to 3 weeks. Watch for possible secondary bacterial involvement of viral lesions. If this occurs, treat with oral anti-staphylococcal antibiotics 3 times daily for 7–10 days.

Herpes zoster can become disseminated. A case is considered disseminated if there exist 20 or more lesions on the skin other than the primarily affected dermatome. These patients are almost always immunosuppressed in some fashion. Pulmonary infection is uncommon.

Post herpetic neuralgia can result after a herpes zoster infection. About $\frac{1}{2}$ of those patients over 50 years old are afflicted with this complication. The patients continue to have pain in the afflicted dermatome even after the rash fully resolves. Most post herpetic neuralgia resolves by 3 months, but about 10% of cases last merely months or even for life.

This complication is difficult to treat effectively. Tricyclic antidepressants and narcotic analgesics are usually sufficient when combined with regular physician visits, support, and proper patient education. If such therapies are not effective, the patient is best managed with referral to a dermatologist for transcutaneous electrical nerve stimulation or counter-irritations. We presume that very early therapy will minimize post-zoster neuralgia.

PEARLS AND PITFALLS

▼ Herpes zoster *is* contagious:

Causes varicella in an individual who has never had varicella in past

Will not cause varicella in individual with history of varicella in past

Will not cause a primary herpes zoster infection in anyone

▼ Occurs in patients with history of varicella

▼ May mimic herpes simplex

▼ Viral cultures useful to distinguish

▼ Tzanck smear not useful to distinguish

▼ If involves ophthalmic dermatome—immediate ophthalmologist referral

▼ If patient in first trimester of pregnancy—inform about possible fetal anomalies

▼ If over 50 years of age—50% chance of post herpetic neuralgia

▼ Oral Valcyclovir useful if started within 96 hours of symptom onset

▶ VARICELLA ZOSTER (CHICKEN POX)

BACKGROUND

This disease is the highly contagious primary infection caused by the DNA varicella zoster virus (VZV). It is almost universally and exclusively seen in children less than 12 years of age. Those (~5%) over the age of 16 usually have a more serious infection with increased likelihood of prodrome (fever, headache, aches, pains, malaise) and complications (pneumonia, encephalitis). The prodrome precedes the rash by approximately 24 hours and is quite uncommon in childhood. At least three viruses other than VZV can cause an eruption on skin that may closely resemble chicken pox. These viral exanthems are discussed in a subsequent section.

The virus is spread via direct transmission and/or airborne droplets. It has a 10–20 day incubation period. As previously noted, the virus is extremely contagious and there is often a history of exposure to an infected individual. Contagion can occur from 2 days before rash until all vesicles have crusted over (usually 7 days).

We now have a highly effective immunization for varicella zoster virus. The potential cost effectiveness in the childhood population is being investigated. Adults who have never had a varicella infection should be immunized due to the increased incidence of severe/complicated infection in this population.

Varicella zoster virus, like all herpes viruses, enter a dormant phase. The virus travels from the skin lesions into the dorsal nerve root of the sensory ganglion. It may be reactivated later in life and cause the development of herpes zoster (shingles).

IN THE CLINIC

Most adults will give a history of headache, low grade fever, aches and pains and severe malaise for 24–48 hours before the eruption of the typical skin changes. Children rarely display such a prodrome and the initial symptoms are the characteristic exanthem.

The pruritic rash consists of widespread lesions which may be few or dense in number. The changes begin as 3–5 mm diameter erythematous macules with centralized, small, yellowish papules. The central papules soon become vesicles and, within 24 hours, have evolved into pustules or broken down to weeping crusts. The vesicular stage of the lesion demonstrates the typical "dew drop on a rose petal" appearance. Lesions begin on the face and move downwards to the trunk, arms, and finally the legs. Lesions can occur anywhere except the hands and the feet. Any mucous membranes can be involved. Lesions on such moist membranes begin as vesicles but quickly proceed to painful ulcerations.

New lesions develop in irregular crops over a 4 day period and almost all lesions are crusted over by 5 days. Contagion continues until all lesions are crusted, at most by 7 days. As previously mentioned, the exanthem of varicella is universally pruritic in nature. Excessive scratching of lesions is almost unavoidable and can lead to significant excoriation, possible scarring, pitting, and an increased likelihood of secondary bacterial pyoderma. Thus, treatment must include measures to minimize the pruritus and prevent scratching.

DIAGNOSIS AND TREATMENT

Clinical suspicion is usually all that is necessary for diagnosis. A Tzanck smear of fluid from a vesicle will demonstrate a herpes virus infection, but it is indistinguishable from the Tzanck smear of a herpes simplex lesion. Viral cultures are very difficult technically, but diagnostic for varicella zoster virus. Tzanck smears and viral cultures are rarely necessary in light of clinical suspicion. If desired, these tests are usually carried out most cost effectively if performed by a dermatologist.

Treatment of varicella in children is usually restricted to symptomatic measures only. Pruritus can be relieved by frequent application of cool water compresses, Aveeno oatmeal baths, or oral antihistamines, such as Atarax, every 8 hours at doses for age and weight. Oral antiviral therapy is rarely necessary.

In adults, more severe infection usually occurs. This population will benefit from oral antiviral therapy, especially if it is initiated within 48 hours of the appearance of the exanthem. Use Valcyclovir at doses of 1 gram 3 times daily for 7 days. Effective doses of Acyclovir are obtainable only with the intravenous medication.

Adult patients may develop concument pneumonia, or encephalitis. These viral complications are most commonly seen in the immunocompromised patient and are further discussed under prognosis, section V of this chapter.

All patients may contract a secondary bacterial pyoderma. Watch for increased redness, exudation, edema, warmth, tenderness, and fever. Treat any pyoderma with a 3 times daily dose of oral anti-staphylococcal antibiotic for 5–7 days. Watch pyodermas closely.

MANAGEMENT

To Manage

▼ Keep all cases in children and all non-immunocompromised adults without pneumonia or encephalitis
▼ Treat children symptomatically for pruritus
▼ Cool tap water compresses PRN
▼ Aveeno oatmeal baths PRN
▼ Oral antihistamines every 8 hours
▼ Treat adults symptomatically as above
▼ If within 48 hours of outbreak, add oral antiviral agent. Either:
  1. Acyclovir by IV route
  2. Valcyclovir 1 gram 3 times a day for 7 days
▼ If secondary pyoderma develops, add an oral anti-staphylococcal antibiotic 3 times daily for 5–7 days.

Send

▼ Infectious disease specialist if possible varicella pneumonia or if mental status changes of possible varicella encephalitis.
▼ Dermatologist with:
  1. All immuno-compromised
  2. Any case requiring Tzanck smear or viral cultures
  3. Necrotic skin lesions

PROGNOSIS

Almost all children recover fully within 7 days of the onset of symptoms. Adults may have the previously discussed prodrome and the uncomplicated infection may cause symptoms that last up to 2 weeks. Again, watch for the complications of varicella pneumonia or encephalitis and refer to or consult with an infectious disease specialist if necessary. In addition, scarring can result if excessive picking and scratching of lesions occurs. The varicella zoster virus can cause fetal anomalies if a pregnant woman is infected during the first trimester of pregnancy.

PEARLS AND PITFALLS

▼ Contagious from time of initial exanthem appearance until all lesions are crusted over approximately 1 week.

▼ Adults may develop varicella pneumonia or encephalitis.

▼ Immuno-compromised patients more likely to have severe, complicated infection.

▼ Patients in 1st trimester of pregnancy have chance of developing secondary fetal anomalies.

▼ Minimizing pruritus will lessen scratching and help prevent both resultant bacterial pyoderma and scarring.

CASE 6.11

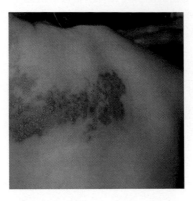

S: A 66-year-old recently retired economics professor presents to your office with complaints of left back and chest pain. He describes the pain as "burning" in nature and denies any radiation. He states the pain began suddenly 4 days ago while he was watching the Home Shopping Network on television and has progressively increased since its onset. He attributes the pain to "sore muscles" because he had been working on cleaning out the garage as per his wife's request the day prior to the symptom's onset. He has been taking Tylenol 1000mg off and on which doesn't help the pain very much. He has been rubbing Ben-gay into the area as well with no relief. He also complains of a headache and feeling very tired for the last 2 days but believes this is because it has been snowing the last 3 days and he has been forced to remain in the house with his wife 24 hours a day. He states he has been feeling "kind of down" since he retired but no more so the last week than he had been previously. He denies any diaphoresis, nausea, shortness of breath or history of such pain in the past. He is a non-smoker and there is no family history of heart disease. He does admit to the development of some pruritus in the same area of the pain just since awakening this morning. He has no further complaints except that he has had to wait 15 minutes before you got into the room and wishes he had never let his wife badger him into coming to see you in the first place.

O: A pleasant man who appears quite tired and whose manner is mildly gruff. This personality change is new in this patient whom you see regularly for health maintenance and acute problem management. His skin demonstrates small (2mm–3mm diameter) erythematous papules in clusters on a red base over the left chest, flank, and back. A mild degree of excoriation is present. No weeping, crusts or other secondary changes are present. When you comment on the rash the patient states "I swear either those were not there this morning or I am developing Alzheimer's Disease which would be just my luck the way life has been going lately." The rest of his skin is without any further abnormality. The rest of his examination is WNL although you do note a somewhat depressed affect which is appropriate for his mood.

A: Herpes Zoster—T6 dermatome; possible depression.

P: Cool water soaks to skin every 4–6 hours

Acetaminophen with Codeine every 4–6 hour for any pain not relived with OTC Tylenol

Oral antihistamine every 8 hours to help relieve the itching

Valacyclovir 1.0 gm orally 3 x each day for 7 days.

Patient education on Herpes Zoster and its possible delayed neuritis.

Start to investigate possible depression symptoms with patient and schedule a follow up visit to further pursue this topic.

PATIENT EDUCATION HANDOUT
HERPES ZOSTER (SHINGLES)

Your rash, pain and itching is from a *virus*.

This virus has been in your system since you had the chicken pox.

It lies asleep after the chicken pox but may reappear to cause the rash you now have.

It may occur again in your life and possibly in a different spot.

If your rash/pain started *in the last 3 days*, your doctor may give you pills to take. Take all medication as instructed, promptly.

You cannot give shingles to anyone else *BUT* you can give a person chicken pox if they have never had it before.

Tell your doctor if you are or think you might be pregnant.

If the pain continues after the rash is gone, contact your physician immediately.

Always call if you have any questions.

▼

PATIENT EDUCATION HANDOUT

VARICELLA ZOSTER (CHICKEN POX)

Try not to scratch your rash—ask your doctor for help if you continue to itch.

Use cool water on wash cloths and towels and apply to itchy area. Repeat as needed to keep itching to a minimum.

Over the counter Benadryl liquid for children and capsules for adults can be used as instructed to decrease the itching.

Calamine lotion, Caladryl lotion, and cortisone creams are not effective in helping itching.

If you develop a cough, shortness of breath, severe headache, chest pain, confusion or any other concerning symptom—call you doctor immediately.

If you have been prescribed a medication, take it as directed until finished.

If you might be pregnant, notify your doctor immediately.

LESS COMMON DISORDERS

▶ BLISTERS AND CHRONIC BULLOUS DISEASES

Many skin diseases present with a blistering component. In this chapter we will focus on those diseases that are primarily blistering or bullous in nature and chronic. Four of the most common types of such disease are pemphigus, pemphigoid, dermatitis herpetiform, and epidermolysis bullosa. These dermatologic diseases often difficult to diagnosis and treat, will be seen in every physician's office because the problem continues over so many years. The best approach to the long-term care of these diseases is discussed here.

▶ PEMPHIGUS

BACKGROUND

Pemphigus is the term employed to describe a set of acute or chronic autoimmune diseases typified by thin-walled blisters on the skin. The disease is rare, seen in both sexes equally, and usually occurs from 40 to 60 years of age. A subpopulation of Jewish individuals of a certain HLA subtype are predisposed to developing pemphigus. The autoimmune disorder leads to IgG antibodies which bind to glycoproteins in the epidermal cell surface. This binding leads to release of proteases and a process known as acantholysis. Acantholysis is the term employed to describe abnormal epidermal cell to cell adhesion. The responsible pemphigus antibodies are regularly found circulating in the affected patient. Pemphigus is believed to be idiopathic, a few cases have been seen as a result of penicillamine and captopril injection.

IN THE CLINIC

Pemphigus usually manifests initially as oral mucous membrane blisters. The overlying flesh-colored vesicle roofs are extremely friable and break down easily. The resultant shallow erythematous erosions are quite painful and are often seen in the posterior oro-pharynx and the nasal mucous membranes, as well as the oral mucosa. An affected patient will often present with sore mouth, a sore throat or dysphagia. Other mucous membrane surfaces may also be affected. These areas include the vagina esophagus, larynx, vulva, penis and rectum.

The mucous membrane findings usually precede the cutaneous rash by up to 6 months. The patients skin demonstrates round-to-oval shaped, discrete flesh-colored bullae and vesicles. Like the mucosal lesions, these bullae/vesicles have overlying roofs that are extremely fragile and often flabby. Thus, they easily rupture with the slightest trauma. As a result the main cutaneous finding is shallow erythematous erosions with significant weeping and crusting. The initial skin lesions arise on the trunk but quickly spread to the face, axillae, groin, scalp predominately with other skin involvement possible as well. The cutaneous erosions are usually not painful, whereas their mucous membrane counterparts can become so painful as to lead to reduced oral intake and possible malnutrition. In addition to the primary epidermal changes a patient may demonstrate secondary weakness, fatigue, weight loss, dysphagic, and epistaxis. These secondary symptoms are primarily a result of the painful oral pemphigus lesions.

DIAGNOSIS AND TREATMENT

Since this autoimmune disorder can prove fatal if untreated, a suspected case should be confirmed via skin biopsy. Choose early small fresh bullae to biopsy if possible. These biopsies should be sent to pathology for diagnosis. It is helpful to collaborate with a dermatologist when biopsying and sending the slides. The specialist can review the slides and employ his/her expertise in the area of dermatopathology to confirm a diagnosis.

Light microscopy will demonstrate the typical acantholytic changes. Direct immunofluorescence of perilesional/unaffected skin will show characteristic IgG deposits in all patients and complement deposits in nearly one half of those affected. In addition, immunofluorescent techniques may be employed on patients serum in an attempt to demonstrate IgG autoantibodies. These are present in the majority of patients and the level is an indicator of the severity of the disease.

Treatment of pemphigus has come a long way in the last 40 years. With the advent of corticosteroid therapy, and, more recently with immunosuppressive adjuncts, the fatality rate has been drastically reduced. Currently, the majority of pemphigus deaths are as a result of therapy—namely drug toxicity. Treatment is with oral prednisone 1–3 mg/kg each day (dependent on disease severity) until no new lesions form. At this point the steroid dose may be tapered carefully to an every other day dosing regimen and/or immunosuppressive therapy may be added concomitantly. Some of the immunosuppressive agents employed in adjunct pemphigus treatment include azathioprine, cyclophosphamide, cyclosporin, and methotrexate. Although these medications have their own toxic side effects, they are still more safe overall than administering high-dose oral corticosteroids alone. Gold salts IM may be valuable in some cases. Collaborate on therapy.

The overall management of pemphigus is time consuming on the part of the physician. Close monitoring of the patient's disease and lab values while on the necessary treatment regimens is essential in reducing morbidity and mortality associated with treatment. Responses are unreliable. Thus, it is often best to refer these patients to a dermatologist who has often managed patients with pemphigus. But, a primary care physician well versed in the diagnosis and treatment of this autoimmune disorder can feel comfortable managing a patient afflicted with this disorder.

MANAGEMENT

To Manage

▼ Keep *only* if well-versed on pemphigus diagnosis and treatment.
▼ Collaboration with a dermatologist at the minimum

Send

We advocate early, prompt referral of all patients.

PROGNOSIS

Pemphigus is a chronic disease with significant morbidity and with a mortality rate of approximately 90% if left untreated. Prognosis improves with early diagnosis and prompt initiation of appropriate therapy. Old age and extensive disease at the time of diagnosis are poor prognostic indicators. Even with appropriate and early treatment, the fatality rate remains at about 10%. Therapy is tedious, requiring constant attention in most cases.

PEARLS AND PITFALLS

▼ Do not delay diagnostic biopsy in any patient with a bullous skin disorder.

▼ Collaborate with a dermatologist.

▼ Remember the importance of patient education in all dermatological disease.

▶ PEMPHIGOID

BACKGROUND

Pemphigoid is another autoimmune disease manifested by bullous skin lesions. Also known as bullous pemphigoid it occurs in a similarly low percentage of the population as ulcer pemphigus. Unlike pemphigus, pemphigoid is usually not manifested until at least 60 years of age and has no genetic predisposition.

This bullous autoimmune disorder also involves circulating autoantibodies. It is these autoantibodies that bind to specific bullous pemphigoid antigens found on stratified squamous epithelium. The specific epithelial structure the antigen is located on is known as a hemidesmosome. These hemidesmosomes are believed to function in the epithelial cell as aids in the binding of the lamina lucida of the basement membrane to the keratinocytic. When the pemphigoid antigen/antibody complex is formed these hemidesmosomes are broken down and the complement system is activated. This initiates a chain of cellular events which eventually involves chemotaxis of neutrophils and eosinophils along with mast cell degranulation. Eventually, the epidermis demonstrates breakdown at the level of the basement membrane. As a result subepidermal bullae form whose transudate consists predominately of eosinophils and mast cells.

IN THE CLINIC

Pemphigoid often begins with a prodromal urticarial vesicular, or papulosquamous rash that is pruritic or "burning." This prodromal phase may last up to 3 months before the characteristic bullous changes appear. The bullae are discrete, oval shaped and tense. They arise from either normal appearing skin or erythematous. Since the lesions arise from the subepidermal layer of the skin they are not covered with a flabby, friable blister roof. Thus, a patient will usually present with numerous intact bullous lesions rather than the predominant erosions typical of pemphigus. The blister fluid ranges in color from clear to pinkish-red. The bullae begin on the trunk but spread quickly to involve the flexor surfaces of the extremities, the axilla and the groin. Mucous membrane lesions can form, but are usually infrequent, appear later, and are mildly painful. These patients lack the constitutional symptoms present in the individual with pemphigus. Pruritus is very common. Subsequent itching is the usual mechanism whereby the thick-roof of the bullae is broken down leaving shallow erosions with typical crusting and weeping. In general, pemphigoid resembles allergic contact dermatitis.

DIAGNOSIS AND TREATMENT

The diagnosis of pemphigoid can be suspected clinically but should be confirmed via biopsy. Again, collaborate with a dermatologist to manage the dermatopathology. Light microscopy will reveal the characteristic subepidermal bullae. Immunofluorescence demonstrates IgG antibodies and complement (L3) deposited in the basement membrane. Although less commonly seen than in pemphigus, pemphigoid will have circulating serum IgG autoantibodies.

Treatment of pemphigoid is less toxic than for pemphigus. In fact, localized mild disease can often be treated with twice daily application of a high-potency topical corticosteroid. If the disease is not mild nor localized systemic corticosteroids must be employed. Initial once a day dosing of 60 to 80 mg of prednisone may be tapered over weeks once the rash improved. Once the patient is at 20 every other day, they can be maintained at this dose. Another option is to add an immunosuppressive agent such as azathioprine, and further taper the prednisone. Dapsone has been used successfully in mild cases where systemic corticosteroid therapy is not possible.

Unlike pemphigus, pemphigoid can be managed effectively in the primary care setting. Collaboration with a dermatologist, especially if not familiar with the treatment course, is helpful.

MANAGEMENT

To Manage

▼ Keep all mild or moderate biopsy proven cases.

▼ Treatment

Localized/mild cases:

Topical high-potency corticosteroid BID

▼ Generalized/moderate cases:

▼ Oral prednisone

60–80 mg every a.m. until controlled

▼ Then taper dose by 10 mg every other day on a 2 week course

▼ Schedule until on strictly every other day dose.

▼ Then taper dose by 10 mg every 2 weeks until

At 20 mg every other day.

▼ Then:

a. Taper by 5 mg every 2 weeks until off

or

b. Add immunosuppressive agent

▼ Mild/generalized case in patient where corticosteroids contraindicated.

▼ Dapsone 100–150 mg a day

▼ Moderate/generalized cases where corticosteroids contra-indicated.

▼ Azathioprine 150 mg every day until remit then 100 mg every day to maintain.

Send

▼ All biopsy proven severe cases

▼ Any case not responsive to above therapy

▼ Any case that worsens

▼ If unfamiliar with therapy

PROGNOSIS

Pemphigoid has a generally good prognosis and has a mortality rate of < 5% even if left untreated. Unfortunately, the disease does occur in the elderly population where concomitant diseases may add to the patients overall risk of death. It is chronic in nature and patients should be educated properly.

PEARLS AND PITFALLS

▼ Even if clinically suspect of pemphigoid—prove the diagnosis with a biopsy.
▼ Collaborate with a dermatologist if any questions.
▼ Educate the patient about their disease—especially its chronicity.
▼ Send all extensive, severe forms to the dermatologist.

▶ DERMATITIS HERPETIFORMIS

BACKGROUND

Dermatitis herpetiformis is a very distressing chronic disorder of the skin. Usually manifested at the age of 30 or 40 years. The disease is known to be twice as common in men as in women. A genetic predisposition to developing dermatitis herpetiformis has been determined with most patients expressing the HLA-38/DZW3 haplotype. Interestingly, most patients with dermatitis herpetiformis also are afflicted with a gluten-sensitive enteropathy and up to 20% of individuals with this rash manifest the enteropathy as small bowel malabsorption.

Details on the exact pathophysiology of the disease are not yet known. Like pemphigus and pemphigoid, this vesicular skin rash demonstrates circulating immune complexes. In this disease the dermatitis herpetiformis specific antibody (IgA) binds to a certain antigen. This IgA antibody—antigen complex is otherwise not well described to date. The relationship of small bowel mucosal membrane and cutaneous epithelium to this same IgA complex is also not yet known. It is known that the complex is somehow involved at the subepidermal layer of the skin. It is at this level that microscopic changes are visualized in biopsied lesions.

IN THE CLINIC

This chronic skin disease presents primarily as erythematous, small, firm-roofed vesicles. These lesions are often mixed with urticarial wheals. The vesicles are extremely pruritic and the patient will scratch at the affected skin which leads to breakdown of the overlying vesicle roof. The resultant shallow erosions with variable secondary weeping and crusting. These vesicles/excoriations/wheels are almost always distributed in a symmetrical fashion over the extensor surfaces of the extremities, the scalp, buttocks, and face. As mentioned earlier the patient may have laboratory evidence of small-bowel malabsorption. But, clinical symptoms of this enteropathy are consistently absent.

DIAGNOSIS AND TREATMENT

A patient suspected of having this disease should undergo biopsy of an early vesicular lesion. Light microscopy demonstrates necrosis, increased numbers of neutrophils and eosinophils, and the presence of a subepidermal vesicles. Immunofluorescence of a biopsy of normal-perilesional areas will demonstrate deposits of linear and granular IgA and complement at the basement membrane. Collaborate with the dermatologist to review the dermatopathology and confirm the pathology.

Also, the presence of subclinical gluten sensitive enteropathy can be seen radiologically via focal areas flattening of small bowel villi. A endoscopic biopsy will confirm the diagnosis.

The disease is usually treated with dapsone 100–200 mg each day until the disease shows improvement. The dose can then be reduced to 25–50 mg each day. Remember to rule out glucose-6-phosphate dehydrogenase deficiency before beginning dapsone therapy. A gluten free diet will either reduce the amount of dapsone necessary for effective therapy or totally alleviate any need for pharmaceutical treatment. Sell the patient on the value of the diet. The disease responds extremely quickly to proper therapy.

MANAGEMENT

To Manage

▼ Keep almost all biopsy proven cases with some collaboration
▼ Treatment:

Dapsone 100–200 mg orally every day until controlled then reduce to 25–50 mg every day and/or

Gluten free diet

▼ Patient education on gluten free diet and chronicity of disease with necessity of long term therapy.

▼ Collaborate with a dermatologist at least once.

Send

If any treatment questions or patient doesn't respond promptly.

PROGNOSIS

As previously noted, dermatitis herpetiformis is a chronic disease. Therapy must be administered long term in order to maintain disease control.

PEARLS AND PITFALLS

▼ Be certain to collaborate with a dermatologist about biopsy results/treatment for all cases.

▼ If clinically suspect, *always* biopsy a lesion to prove this disease as the diagnosis.

▶ EPIDERMOLYSIS BULLOSA

Epidermolysis bullosa is the term employed to describe a collection of over a dozen specific types of blistering skin diseases. All of these dermatologic abnormalities are a result of a hereditary abnormality in the epidermal to dermal junction. Although each separate disease has its own clinical appearance, histological changes, pathophysiology, and mode of inheritance, all epidermolysis bullosa patients are afflicted with easily blistering skin. Their cutaneous and mucous membrane surfaces are quite easily affected by even the slightest trauma to induce blister formation. All of the forms of epidermolysis bullosa demonstrate the blisters at the subepidermal layer. This set of skin disorders are quite rare and will not be discussed in any further deal. If a patient presents with a rash of where blister/erosions predominate suspect epidermolysis bullosa. Biopsy of early lesions should always be performed to confirm the diagnosis. Treatment varies depending on the type of epidermolysis bullosa diagnosed and should be tailored based on the biopsy results. Always collaborate with a dermatologist when treating these patients.

CASE 7.1

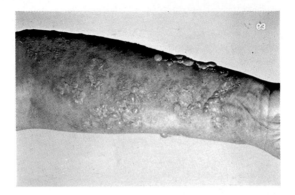

S: An 83-year-old white female patient of your partner presents to your clinic in Tinley Park, Illinois while he is on vacation. She complains of a 2 week history of a concerning rash on her abdomen, arms and legs. She states the rash was red and "hive-like" for the first 10 days, but has become covered with blisters over the past 4 or 5 days. She does admit that the entire time the lesions have been extremely pruritic and she has had to use antihistamines to control the itch. Even this medication has not been totally relieving. Otherwise she is an exceptionally healthy patient who has no significant medical illnesses and is on no medications.

O: A slight, but well-nourished, elderly white female who appears younger than her stated age. She has stable vital signs and is not febrile. Her skin demonstrates poorly-marginated erythematous plaques over the extensor surfaces of her arms and legs as well as over her abdomen. There are multiple clear fluid-filled vesicles and bulla overlying the plaques. A few erosions are present along with a moderate amount of excoriation. The rest of her skin is without abnormality. A complete physical examination reveals no further pertinent findings.

LAB: Chem 20—within normal limits

CBC—Slight increase in eosinophils but otherwise within normal limits

Sedimentation Rate—within normal limits

A: Bullous Skin Disease—history and physical lead towards a diagnosis of Bullous Pemphigoid

P: Immediate phone consultation with and referral to a dermatologist. Do not hesitate to refer patients with bullous skin lesions.

PATIENT EDUCATION HANDOUT
BLISTERS AND CHRONIC BULLOUS DISEASES

Your doctor has diagnosed your disease as_____.
_____

    These skin diseases are very hard to pronounce but are well known to your physician.

    You are asked to begin the medication called

_____.

Your should take this medication as follows:

_____.

    Your doctor may ask you to see a dermatologist (a skin doctor) to help to treat your disease.

    Your doctor has the other instructions as outlined here below:_____
_____
_____
_____
_____

▶BURNS AND FROSTBITE

▶ BURNS

BACKGROUND

The most common burn is sunburn. Sunburn has been thoroughly discussed in the heliosis chapter of this book. It can be viewed as a first degree thermal burn.

Patients who sustain cutaneous burns will often present with constitutional symptoms. The more severe the burn the more toxic the patient. A sunburn can induce fever, chills, and malaise. A third degree burn can cause hypovolemic shock and these patients usually require long-term hospitalization.

Other therapy for first and second degree burns includes: analgesia, aspirin daily at doses of 650 mg every 4–6 hours is the most effective choice. If a child under 16 years old, ibuprofen per age/weight may be used every 6–8 hours. Pruritus is well controlled with oral antihistamines every 6–8 hours.

MANAGEMENT

To Manage

- ▼ Keep all 1st and 2nd degree burns.
- ▼ Treatment:
  1st degree—Apply antibiotic gel or petroleum jelly to area.
- ▼ *No* topical anesthetics.
- ▼ Good wound care
- ▼ Open-to-air/no dressings necessary.
  2nd degree—Clean wound thoroughly.
- ▼ Debride if necessary
- ▼ Silver sulfadine—apply thick layer
- ▼ Burn dressing with padding and elastic support—change daily.
- ▼ Recheck wound after OD until healing well and decreased risk of pyoderma.

Send

All third degree burns to burn team at appropriate facility. Stabilize first.

▶ FROSTBITE

BACKGROUND

Frostbite is another strong irritant contact dermatitis. The vast majority of frostbite arises from poor preparation for cold weather conditions. Remember that wind and moisture will significantly intensify the potential cutaneous injury inflicted by cold termperatures. Extremities and other areas with poor blood supply are the most easily injured. In a brisk cold wind at zero centigrade, just going out without a hat to scrape off the car windows can result in frostbite of ears and face. Commonly injured sites include the ears, nose, fingertips, and toes. Male joggers are at risk for frostbite of their genitalia if they exercise outdoors in winter weather. Winter outdoor activity at high altitudes is a common predictor for possible frostbite. Patients with cold urticaria or cryogloblininema will have atypical responses even to minor cold injury.

Skin does not freeze easily. A temperature of $-20°C$ or below for a prolonged time period is required for cutaneous cold injury. Structures potentially affected include the subcutaneous tissue, bursa, tendons and bone as well as the skin. At about 20°C all cellular metabolism stops. Protein and enzymes in affected cells denature and extracellular ice crystals form. Water is thus extracted from the cells and dehydration with possible necrosis occurs. In the epidermis, most of the damage is due to the extracellular ice crystal formation. In the dermis, the low temperature leads to vascular damage and subsequent thrombosis, dessication, and destabilization of protein-lipid-glycan colloids.

Frost bite also can occur from some sprays, from dry ice, and from handling frozen materials. The clinical appearance of frostbite varies depending on the depth of the injury, the skin is usually brightly erythematous and edematous with patches of white or hypopigmentation. Necrosis does occur and can be quite severe. The patient complains of burning, hypesthesia, or possibly from numbness.

Treatment of frostbite includes rapid rewarming in a circulating water bath at 39–44°C. Avoid friction massage as it often worsens the injury. Rewarming as above is quite effective and frozen tissue without necrosis re-vascularizes and fully recovers within 48 hours. Any tissue that continues to demonstrate necrosis after 48 hours may require surgical debridement. Scaring, paraesthesia and hyperhidrosis may remain after treatment.

MANAGEMENT

To Manage

- ▼ Keep all cases
- ▼ Treatment
  Rapid rewarming in circulating water bath at 38–44 °C
- ▼ NO FRICTION MASSAGE
- ▼ After 48 hours if necrosis present—thorough debridement
- ▼ Patient education
- ▼ Proper clothing; watch time exposure
- ▼ Increased likelihood with wind, moisture-laden clothing, and altitude

Send

- ▼ Only if large areas of debridement necessitate intricate surgery.
- ▼ If atypical reaction

CASE 7.2

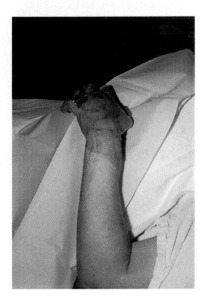

S: A 22-year-old white male presents to the emergency room where you work in New Orleans, Louisiana. Apparently he had been preparing a crawfish boil with a group friends on his softball team when the pot of boiling water was accidently knocked over. Unfortunately, the hot water (and a few "bugs") landed on his left arm and hand. Although the extremity was immediately placed under cold running water he decided he had better come in and have it looked at by a doctor. He admits that the burned skin is extremely painful now that the anesthetic effect of the margarita he had been drinking is starting to wear off. He has no history of prior skin disease or other medical illness and is taking no medications.

O: A pleasant and jovial young white male who appears his stated age, is well nourished and is in no acute distress. The skin over the left arm demonstrates a well-demarcated patch of bright-red erythema from the left wrist extending distally over the dorsum of the left hand. There are multiple clear-fluid filled blisters and a few erosions over the area of skin change. The entire patch of abnormal skin is exquisitely tender to even the lightest palpation. The rest of the skin is without abnormality. The remainder of the physical examination is entirely unremarkable.

A: Second-degree burn to the left upper extremity.

P: Cool water compresses as needed for pain. Silvadene cream applied liberally to area twice each day followed by careful dressing with a non-adherent bandage. The burn should be rechecked in 24 to 48 hours to ensure proper healing. The patient should be warned about possible secondary pyoderma and should be instructed to return immediately if such changes should occur.

PATIENT EDUCATION HANDOUT
BURNS

You have been diagnosed with a skin burn by your physician.

Doctors can "grade" a burn from a First Degree which is not too bad to a Third Degree which is very serious. A Second Degree burn is worse than a First Degree burn but not as bad as a Third Degree Burn. Your burn is a _____ Degree Burn.

Your doctor may ask you to take some medicine to help treat your burn. He or She suggests the medicines that are checked below:

❏ Aspirin—325mg tablets—take 2 of these every 4 to 6 hours as you need to for pain. If you cannot take aspirin please tell your doctor so they can give you a different pain medicine.

❏ Ibuprofen should be used in children under the age of 16 rather than aspirin. Your doctor wants you to give your child the following dose _____.

❏ Benadryl is available over the counter at most grocery stores and pharmacies. It is also called Diphenhydramine. We use this medicine to help with the swelling and the itching of your burn. It is available in a liquid or in a pill form. Your doctor recommends you take the following dose _____ _____.

❏ _____ _____

Sometimes your doctor will ask you to use a medicine you smooth onto the surface of the burned skin. He or She suggests the medicines that are checked below:

❏ Antibiotic ointments are available over the counter. You should put this on the area burned two times each day to prevent an infection.

❏ Silver sulfadine is a thick white pasty cream that helps to soothe your burn. You should use this medicine two times a

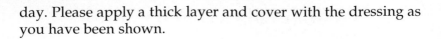

day. Please apply a thick layer and cover with the dressing as you have been shown.

❒ _____
_____.

You should follow up with your doctor as he or she has asked.

PATIENT EDUCATION HANDOUT
FROSTBITE

You have been diagnosed with having skin that has been what is called "Frostbite." It is a disease caused by your skin being in the cold for too long a time.

Your doctor has asked you to take the following medication for pain. Be certain to take it as he or she has asked you to:

_____

_____

It is important to dress the right way when you are going out in the cold weather. Always wear enough clothes and warm clothes. Wear two pairs of socks if you plan to be out in the cold for a long time. The longer you are out in the cold the more likely you are to get a frostbite.

The chances of frostbite increase with any wind, at high altitudes (especially skiing), and if your clothes are at all wet. Cold and wet together add up to frostbite if you are not careful and warm up soon or change out of wet clothes.

If you have any questions be sure to ask your doctor.

▶ DERMATOLOGIC EMERGENCIES

Certain uncommon groups of skin diseases may be counted as true emergencies. Not only should the primary care physician consult immediately with the dermatologist on these cases, but the prior agreement ought to be that almost every case will be managed collaboratively in person, immediately, and with the consultant. This precaution recognizes these cases are deceptive and difficult and that laboratory tests, especially selective biopsies, may need to be done and interpreted without delay. Immediate treatment may be essential. Finally, important errors may be avoided by proper planning and management of the situation. Three groups are: 1) New and numerous bulla, 2) Necrosis of the skin, either focal or in sheets, 3) Generalized acute inflammation of skin, such as vast numbers of pustules, or erythrodermatitis, or massive exudations.

NEW BULLA

Any sudden, unexplained eruption of numerous new cutaneous bullae is an emergency. The most common acute disease in this group is bullous erythema multiforme. Notice involvement of lips, mouth, or eyes. Many blisters may contain blood, in the worst cases, look for target lesions on the hands and over joints. Involvement of eyes, mouth and genitals is seen early. Immediate care in a hospital burn unit may be appropriate after tests and biopsies to establish the diagnosis. Steroids are seldom beneficial, debridement should be restrained and cautious. Every effort to establish a cause (often, in adults, a drug reaction) should be made quickly. Plasmapheresis may be useful.

Other considerations for acute severe bullous diseases would be pemphigoid, pemphigus or, rarely, a few other rare conditions.

NECROSIS OF SKIN

One can afford to lose very little skin before the risk of dying increases quickly. Thermal burns can necrose skin, and pose to most common cause of death from acute skin necrosis.

Necrosis can be focal, as from necrotizing infections, usually streptococcal, for from vascular occlusion, often as part of diabetes.

Emboli can cause focal necrosis. A anomalous coagulation can produce thromboses that necrose the skin. Vasculitis can be necrotic. The brown recluse spider bite and certain snake bites can necrose the skin focally. Because the difference between a potentially fatal necrotizing streptococcal infection and a more benign necrotic spider bite many be ambiguous early. It is urgent to obtain an accurate diagnosis urgently. A tissue diagnosis for bacteria is the standard.

Toxic epidermal necrolysis is a true emergency. It is often fatal, especially so when physicians are slow to respond. Almost always, this illness is caused by a drug, most often a sulfa, an anti-epileptic, or an NSAID. Systemic steroids are counterindicated because infections the most common cause of death. If the correct diagnosis is made early (by biopsy and examination) then the use of cyclosporin can prevent vast further risks.

GENERALIZED DEEP INFLAMMATION

The sudden appearance of large fields of identical small pustules, quickly extending to 20% or more of the body surface within hours, is the typical course of pustular psoriasis. Known as the von Zumbusch syndrome, this alarming eruptions is accompanied by malaise, fever, a large leukocytosis, and electrolyte dysfunctions. Managed poorly, the fatality rate may be almost 50%.

Acute erythrodermatitis may result from drug hypersensitivity and, although the prognosis is much better than generalized pustular diseases, the situations urgent. This disorder is caused by drugs such as gold salts and antiseizure medication.

An acute disseminated eczema may occur in severe allergy to nickel (and to other allergens) that resembles erythrodermatitis, but is a more shallow inflammation. Discomfort may be extreme and merit emergency management.

PURPURA

Purpura are very common if one includes bug bites, trauma, coughing, vomiting and positional (hanging upside down) strains. Next most common are "toxic purpura" which occur in many patients, from merely being ill, often with common infections such a influenza, or streptococcal pharyngitis. Toxic purpura may be alarming after envenomations by spiders, wasps, bees or snakes. Localized "easy bruising" purpura occur whenever the dermal supports for blood vessels are defective as in advanced age or photodamage or scurvy, Cushing's syndrome, amyloidosis and a series of hereditary disorders. All of these are harmless purpura.

Platelet deficiencies cause a scattering of tiny petechia, while clotting factor defects usually cause excessive large-size bruising. In all of these forms, the bleeding into skin is *macular*. When the purpura are palpable, we can presume a sustained inflammation around the blood vessels, and hence we diagnose "classic purpura," a more concerning kind, as caused by major diseases. Among these diseases are the rheumatic series (lupus, rheumatoid arthritis, Periarteritis, Sjogren's) and the embolic series (cryoglobulinemia, septic emboli, cholesterol, artefactual, impure IV drugs and transfusions). In addition, consider hypersensitivity reactions such as anaphylaxis, erythema multiforme, Henoch-Schonlein, and some other eruptive skin diseases. Finally, drugs have a wide range of mechanisms able to produce purpura; consider heparin, Coumadin, aspirin, sulfa-like drugs, and NSAIDs. If purpura are accompanied by necrosis, bulla, unusual pain or pigment, scarring or sclerosis, arrange consultation. Do a thorough evaluation.

CASE 7.3

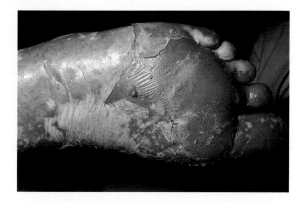

S: A 48 year old white male presents to your clinic for the first time. He is concerned about "blisters" that have developed on his feet and hands over the last 24 hours. He sates the rash is non-tender and denies any associated pruritus. He admits to malaise and mild nausea which began about 6 hours after he first noticed the rash. When asked about his past medical history he admits to having had psoriasis and asthma for many years. Apparently, he developed a upper respiratory infection one week ago which led to significant cough and shortness of breath not helped by his inhalers alone. He visited his normal physician 3 days prior to today's visit. This physician placed him on an oral corticosteroid taper which he has been taking as instructed. He is otherwise healthy and has no other medical illnesses.

O: A well-nourished pale appearing male who seems his stated age. His vital signs are stable and he is not febrile. The skin over his feet and hands demonstrate confluent patches of erythema with overlying pustules, a significant degree of peeling, and a few erosions. The extensor surface of his knees and elbows as well as his buttocks have well-demarcated erythematous plaques with large silver white scale. A piece of scale when pulled off leaves a small spot of blood in its place. There is no excoriation. Otherwise the skin is within normal limits. His nose demonstrates mildly boggy mucous membranes and copious clear nasal drainage. He has clear post nasal drainage as well. His lung sounds are distant but his lung fields are otherwise clear to auscultation. The rest of his physical examination is unremarkable.

A: 1. Pustular skin disease—possible pustular psoriasis
2. Classic psoriasis
3. Upper respiratory infection

P: Immediate phone consultation with a dermatologist and prompt referral for this possible dermatologic emergency.

PATIENT EDUCATION HANDOUT
DERMATOLOGIC EMERGENCIES

No appropriate handout for this section. This chapter is meant to outline those skin diseases that require your patients receive immediate attention from a dermatologist if one is available in your area. If there is no such dermatologist at your disposal than these diseases should not wait. Either refer to a more in depth text of dermatology for specific treatment regimens or transport the patient to a facility where a dermatologist is available and willing to take over their care.

▶ DRUG RASHES

The use of any medication can induce cutaneous eruption. Such an eruption can be termed as "drug rash." These skin lesions arise as an undesirable side effect of the administered medication and will vary in their presentation. Some drug reactions are caused by one or another kind of allergy. Many drug reactions are not allergic, but are due to activations of normal bodily mechanisms such as melanin synthesis or cornification, or to the triggering of inflammatory systems. The exact appearance of a drug rash and the presence of absence of any systemic findings depends on the exact causative agent, the patient's degree of hypersensitivity, the presence of any previous illness or skin disease, and whether or not other drugs are being administered concomitantly. Possible cutaneous changes induced by medication include exanthems, urticaria, angioedema, acne erythroderma, ichthyosis, hyper pigmentation, palpable purpura, focal necrosis, and toxic epidermal necrosis (Table 7.1).

Those medications that lead to two or more cases of drug rash per one thousand patients administered deserve close attention and patient education when prescribed. Examples of drugs that commonly lead to cutaneous side effects include sulfa, ampicillin, synthetic penicillin, cephalosporins, NSAID's, antiseizure medications such as phenytoin, whole blood, and platelets. (Table 7.2). Approximately three percent of all hospital inpatients have some form of skin eruption as a result of a medication they are being given.

The vast majority of drug side effects are minor transient and limited to a mild skin eruption. These rashes are most commonly exanthems and urticaria. Such mild drug rashes require symptomatic

TABLE 7.1 ▼ Possible Types of Skin Change as a Result of Drug Ingestion

Cutaneous Change	Chapter
Exanthem	7
Urticaria	6
Angioedema	6
Erythroderma	6
Hyper pigmentation	7
Toxic epidermal necrosis	8
Palpable purpura	8

TABLE 7.2 ▼ Drugs Commonly Leading to Cutaneous Reaction

Medication	Incidence
Trimethoprim—Sulfa	6/1000
Ampicillin	6/1000
Penicillin	3/1000
Cephalosporins	3/1000
NSAIDs	2–3/1000
Whole blood	4/1000
Platelets	2–3/1000

treatment as well as discontinuation of the offending drug. Once the responsible medication is stopped the patient's cutaneous lesions usually resolve in 2–3 days. Symptomatic treatment of any associated pruritus or pain should be provided. Be certain to let the patient know about their drug "allergy." Also place a prominent notation in the patient's chart.

If a patient has a significant hypersensitivity to a medication, the urticarial skin changes may be associated with angioedema or even possible anaphylaxis. Angioedema has the potential to be life threatening if accompanied by systemic symptoms, or airway compromise. Anaphylaxis is always a medical emergency and these patients should be brought to an appropriate medical facility once stabilized.

Various medications can lead to hyperpigmentation of a patient's skin. The most common etiologic drug are oral contraceptives. Unfortunately, such pigmentation changes do not universally resolve once the offending agent is discontinued. Often patients must undergo the use of azelaic acid, chemical peels, or laser therapy to improve the cosmetic appearance of hyper pigmentation. Also, the affected individual must avoid sunlight or UVB exposure without adequate sunscreen protection. If the patients treated skin is not protected from UVB rays the pigmentary abnormalities often reoccur or worsen.

Other drugs such as methotrexate may cause hair loss or nail dystrophies. Oral corticosteroids may induce acne or purpura or striae. Injectable gold salts or minocycline or amiodarone may pigment the skin. Diuretic drugs may reduce sweating rates so as to predispose elderly patients to overheating. Some drugs, such as niacin, can induce an ichthyosis-like change. A large variety of rare reactions to drugs have been reported and require the physician's attention.

TEN, palpable purpura, and erythroderma can all present as possible dermatologic emergencies and should be approached with the appropriate degree of physician concern and collaboration. If the cutaneous changes are extensive or accompanied by systemic symptoms such as fever, hypo-hypertension, joint pain, gastrointestinal disturbances, malaise the drug reaction is severe and may worsen rapidly. The insulting agent responsible for the patient's reaction should be determined quickly and immediately discontinued. Even without systemic symptoms, skin lesions such as bulla, extensive pustules, necrosis, or purpura should raise physician concern. Always be certain to collaborate at a minimum when managing these patients. Prompt dermatological referral is often recommended as a result of collaboration and is quite appropriate in the vast majority of cases. Seminars on the management of drug eruptions are worthwhile, as the subject is both medically challenging and beneficial to patients.

CASE 7.4

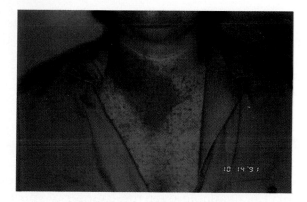

S: A 54 year old female presents to an urgent care clinic with a 12 hour history of a generalized rash. She states the rash is quite itchy and denies any history of such a rash in the past. She denies any SOB, dysphagia, or other complaints. She is usually a healthy individual and visits her physician for routine health maintenance only. When performing a review of systems she does admit to a week-long history of generalized aching muscles. She states she has just joined a health club 2 weeks prior and her personal trainer has been pushing her activity level leading to the generalized soreness of her muscles. When questioned about medications she denies any regular use, but does state she has been using some samples of Voltaren on and off over the last week. This drug was given to her by a neighbor who is an RN at a local orthopedic clinic. She otherwise has a benign past medical history and review of systems.

O: A well-fed, well nourished white female. Vital signs stable. The skin shows a erythematous papular rash over the skin surface of the trunk, upper extremities, and lower extremities. The face appears to be spared and the chest appears to be the most involved. There is evidence of excoriation but it is quite mild, otherwise there exists no further secondary change. The rest of the examination is unremarkable including a full musculoskeletal examination.

A: Drug eruption secondary to NSAID use.

P: Discontinue use of NSAID's and warn against her future use of these medications.
Cool water baths with colloidal oatmeal as needed.
Oral antihistamine every 6–8 hours to alleviate pruritus.

PATIENT EDUCATION HANDOUT
DRUG RASHES

Your doctor has diagnosed your rash as being caused by a medication you have taken. This rash means that you are **allergic** to the medicine.

Many medicines can cause a rash. Your doctor believes your rash is caused by _____.

Stop taking this medicine right away.

Let all your doctors and anyone who prescribes you medication know you are **allergic** to this medicine.

Your doctor has asked you to take the following medications—take only the ones with the box that is checked in front of them.

❐ Benadryl is available over the counter at most grocery stores and pharmacies. It is also called Diphenhydramine. We use this medicine to help with the swelling and the itching of your rash. It is available in a liquid or in a pill form. Your doctor recommends you take the following dose _____

_____

❐ You have been prescribed a steroid pill to take by mouth. Take the medicine as prescribed and as follows_____

_____

Be sure to take all the medicine. Do not stop the medicine until it is all gone or your rash may come back.

❐ You can take baths with Aveeno Oatmeal to help with the itching. It is at most pharmacies and can help out a lot.

❐ Keep your skin moist with a cream or lotion such as _____. This product may be used as often as you need to. The drier your skin is the more it will itch.

❐ _____

_____

Call your doctor if the rash worsens, if you get a fever or if you have any questions.

If you have problems breathing, chest pain or trouble swallowing go to the emergency room right away.

▶ EPITHELIAL SKIN CANCER

The common epithelial skin cancers are of two types—squamous cell carcinoma and basal cell carcinoma. These common neoplasms are different from melanoma in regards to their morbidity. Squamous cell carcinoma (SCC) and basal cell carcinoma (BCC) are malignancy and may lead to morbidity, but, their local spread is quite slow and they rarely metastasize. Thus, they are usually discovered early enough to allow removal prior to the recurrence of significant morbidity. BCC and SCC will be discussed separately below.

▶ BASAL CELL CARCINOMA

BACKGROUND

The BCC is the most common form of skin cancer seen in the clinic. In 1996, over 400,000 patients were newly diagnosed with a BCC. These skin cancers are seen most commonly in men over the age of 40, although, women and those patients < 40 years old can be afflicted. As with melanoma, BCC occurs in sun damaged skin in the fair-skinned light-eyed populations who have a large cumulated exposure to sunlight/UVR over the course of their lives. Truly black-skinned people almost never have epitheliomas. Thus, it is understandable that BCC is seen most commonly in warm, sunny climates on those fair-skinned patients who have had life long exposure to sunlight-farmers, roofers, lifeguards, etc. BCC occur on skin that is bare to the sunlight such as the face, neck, shoulders, back and forearms. There exists rare autosomal dominant disease termed the basal cell nevus syndrome where multiple BCC occur starting in childhood on any skin surface independent of its history of exposure to sunlight. Other risk factors for developing BCC include a history of ionizing radiation exposure and a family history of BCC in youth.

BCC develops due to the UVB form of sunlight or artificial light sources (such as tanning beds). In those patients with little or no (albinos) melanocytic protection, and certain genetic predispositions the UVB light will cause secondary DNA changes. The affected DNA can be at the level of the dermis as well as the epidermis. Also, the UVB light can be immunosuppressive. Thus, the DNA abnormalities along with lowered cellular immunity lead to skin cell injury and inability to repair the damage. These two factors is what allows a BCC to appear and the malignancy to enlarge.

BCC will grow locally due to the factors noted previously but cannot actually metastasize. The lack of metastatic ability stems from the reliance the tumor cells have on the BCC stroma for growth. If a tumor cell is not at the site of the BCC it cannot survive and will die. This stroma growth dependent phenomena disallows metastasis of BCC to occur, with only rare exceptions.

IN THE CLINIC

The clinical appearance of a BCC can vary but all of these lesions are characterized by poor healing, pruritus, and friability. Patients often tell of seeing flecks of blood on their pillow or towel. The far majority of these cancers are of the *nodulo ulcerative* form. Nodulo ulcerative BCC are roundish shaped, translucent to pink colored papules or nodules. They may have an overlying pearly hue. Lesions are usually singular, discrete, and well marginated. Close inspection often reveals a few telangiectasias and palpation demonstrates a typically hard, rubbery possibly cystic, feel. If left alone, nodulo ulcerative BCC will enlarge, erode, and eventually ulcerate. The typical ulcer is superficial with "heaped-up" or "rolled" margins.

Unlike its previously described cousin, *superficial* BCC does not erode. Rather, these erythematous patches of skin cancer enlarge superficially and can become 2–3 cm in diameter. They often have a degree of secondary scale, are multiple in number, and are usually found on the extremities. Pigmented BCC are not pearly white or pink. Rather, these skin cancers are dark blue to black in color and afflict the dark skinned population. Otherwise, they are clinically very similar to the nodulo ulcerative variant. Finally, BCC can be *morphea form*. This type of BCC is noticeable for its aggressive invasion of the normal, surrounding skin. It appears quite like scar tissue, poorly marginated, whitish-yellow, and indurated. Very few BCC are of the morphea form type, but these are the most dangerous.

DIAGNOSIS AND TREATMENT

The diagnoses of BCC and SCC are clinical with histopathological confirmation. It is best to examine a patients skin at every annual health-maintenance visit. It is in this setting the majority of epithelial tumors are discovered. If a lesion suspicious of BCC or SCC is discovered, perform a shave biopsy of the abnormal area. An epithelial lesion > 2 cm in diameter is not easily shaved for biopsy. In this case, multiple punch biopsies from various sites of affected tissue are possible. Label your specimens precisely. When sending the specimen to pathology, you should collaborate with a dermatologist to review the slides and enable proper dermatopathological diagnosis.

If you discover a questionable skin lesion that is < 0.5 cm in diameter, and is not in the high-risk area of the face it is appropriate to watch the lesion. A 3 month recheck must be performed to follow-up on the skin abnormality. At this time the lesion may be biopsied if it has taken on a more characteristic appearance. It is also possible to arrange a single consultation with your dermatologist in the case of a small, questionable lesion. Often a simple visit can save the excessive biopsy against the low cost of a consultation. The overall goal is to balance the high costs of such management in order to save money, time and worry for all parties involved by avoiding excessive biopsy of benign skin lesions. Review your collected cases together in quality assessment.

Treatment of BCC and SCC is similar and will be discussed together. These epithelial skin tumors are treated with cryosurgery, primary excision with closure, electrodesiccation with curettage or Mohs (Cutaneous Micrographic Surgery). Any recurrent BCC or SCC should be immediately referred for Mohs surgery. This microsurgical technique is labor-intensive and must be performed by a properly trained physician with the appropriate equipment. Other epitheliomas that require immediate referral for Mohs include those tumors in the high risk areas of the face—eyelids, nose, perinasal folds, ears, and upper cheeks. These areas of the face all have very thin amounts of subcutaneous tissue and stroma overlying cartilage and bone. Thus, local spread of SCC and BCC may include these underlying structures and removal can involve disfigurement.

If an epithelial skin cancer is superficial and small it may be treated with cryotherapy and close follow-up. Such small BCC and SCC may also be treated with electrodesiccation and curettage if the equipment is available. This technique is performed three times and like cryotherapy, should not be performed on morpheic BCC. Wide elliptical excision of any SCC/BCC that is < 2.0 cm in diameter can undergo primary closure with cosmetic success. The excised tissue must be sent for pathological determination that appropriates margins of normal tissue are present. The future treatment of BCC and SCC holds promise if newer techniques such as CO_2 lasers, immunotherapy, and chemotherapy continue to be improved. Develop an agreed upon plan for your group.

MANAGEMENT

To Manage

▼ Keep: any biopsy confirmed BCC that:

1. Is not a recurrence
2. Is not in the high-risk facial area
3. Is not > 2 cm in diameter
4. Is not a morphea form variant of BCC

▼ Treat:

1. Small (< 0.5 cm) superficial lesions with cryotherapy or electrodesiccation and curettage.
2. Large lesions (0.5 cm–2 cm diameter) with elliptical excision and primary closure.

▼ Educate:

1. Importance of follow-up visits to monitor any recurrence of a lesion.
2. Liberal use of sunscreen
3. Return between annual check-ups if any new lesions develop
4. High risk factors for developing BCC/SCC discussed

Send

▼ Any biopsy proven BCC that:

1. Is recurrent (send for Mohs surgery)
2. Is in the high-risk facial area (to Mohs)
3. Is > 2 cm in diameter (excision with complex closure)
4. Is a morphea form variant (to Mohs)

▼ Any questionable lesion < 0.5 cm in diameter for second opinion.

PROGNOSIS

As mentioned earlier in this chapter the metastasis rate of BCC is very low (< 0.3%). These locally invasive epithelial skin cancers if removed fully have a very low associated morbidity/mortality rate. Unfortunately, tumor cells are often left behind after initial treatment and the skin cancer reoccurs locally. Thus, the patient must be followed up yearly to recheck the skin for any possible recurring lesions. Also, nearly 50% of all patients diagnosed with a BCC will have another such lesion develop later in life. The high expectation for another primary BCC occurring is another factor which that requires close follow-up of these patients.

PEARLS AND PITFALLS

▼ Patients at high risk for BCC:

1. Those with outdoor professions and fair skin
2. Sunbathers
3. Persons who frequent UV tanning beds
4. Family history of skin cancer/BCC
5. Those living in warm, sunny climates

▼ At each visit recognize and record:

1. Any small (0.5 cm in diameter) questionable lesions with scheduled recheck in 3 months.
2. Patient skin type
3. Risk factors
4. Family history of skin cancers

▼ Stress patient education:

1. Sunscreen use—liberally/frequently
2. Self-skin examination
3. Importance of compliance with follow-up visits

▼ Epitheliomas grow slowly in the elderly patient population. If an aged individual has poor health or poor financial resources it is not necessary to approach these lesions aggressive, or to treat them at all.

▼ Pigmented BCC can mimic melanoma in the more dark skinned population. Always *punch biopsy* those lesions which you suspect could be melanoma. Proceed with proper management after the diagnosis is pathological confirmed and discussed with your dermatologist.

▼ Remember to collaboratively approach unusual clinical problems and all histopathological diagnosis.

▶ SQUAMOUS CELL CARCINOMA

BACKGROUND

Although SCC is less common than is BCC, the former accounts for a far greater percentage of epithelioma morbidity and mortality. The reason for this fact is a SCC's ability to metastasize. A SCC can spread both regionally and to distant locations such as the brain, bone, or liver. SCC is most frequently seen in men and usually appears after the age of 55 years old.

This malignancy involves changes of the epidermal cell layer and can arise from mucous membranes as well as the skin. The tumor can be graded histologically according to the degree of differentiation its component cells have undergone. In general, the more well-differentiated the lesion the lower its grade. Staging of SCC is based on its level of spread. The prognosis of a particular SCC is dependent on its histologic grade and clinical stage. SCC-in-situ is restricted to the epithelium only. These abnormal epidermal cells have the ability to invade the local dermis and later any underlying bone, muscle or cartilage. If left untreated, a SCC may metastasize regionally and remotely via the lymphatics or the blood.

As with other skin cancers, SCC has a variety of risk factors. The most common etiology is chronic over exposure to UVR—natural or artificial. Thus, like BCC, SCC is more common in sunny climates and those individuals whose occupation requires outdoor work. Fair skinned individuals who burn easily and rarely tan have the skin types at risk for developing these epitheliomas. Although lightly pigmented skin is a risk factor for sunlight induced SCC, dark skinned individuals may display this skin cancer due to another etiology. Other common etiologies for SCC include those listed in 7.3. Thus, the exact etiology of a specific SCC can be carried and a thorough history and physical must always be performed before assuming the patient's sole risk factor is UVR.

IN THE CLINIC

Actinic keratosis are known commonly as "precancerous" skin lesions. Although sun induced skin damage is a precursor to SCC development; and actinic keratosis is one example of such a poikiloderma. The term "precancer" remains a misname. In fact, only about 0.1–1% of all actinic keratosis transform into SCC. The most worrisome actinic keratosis are those 1 cm in diameter or larger lesions that are indurated and feel "deep" when palpated.

SCC is like its basal cell "cousin" in its lack of homogeneity between lesions. Almost all SCC begin as isolated keratotic plaques or papules but that is where the similarity of features ends. These lesions are most notable for their persistence and slow growth. Any such lesion that is present for more than 1–2 months should be suspect for SCC.

The clinical appearance of a specific SCC is dependent on its depth, its location, and degree of differentiation. Often a biopsy report will refer to a suspect lesion as SCC in-situ. These lesions do not involve skin layers deeper than the epidermis, but the later displays full-thickness changes. In-situ SCC are usually macular scaly, well demarcated and slow growing. Two common types of SCC in-situ are Bowen's disease and erythroplasia of Queyrat. Bowen's disease is a single lesion of in-situ SCC that may be found on any skin. Areas of skin exposed to sunlight may develop Bowen's disease. It can also be caused by arsenic in which case the lesion may be found on skin normally protected from UVR. Erythroplasia of Queyrat is an in-situ SCC that develops on the glans, corona, or prepuce of the penis. Seen most commonly in uncircumcised patients this cancer is more aggressive than other intra epithelial SCC.

Any in-situ SCC may become invasive in nature. These skin cancers vary in clinical presentation with the degree of differentiation they posses. Highly differentiated SCC are usually quite well keratinized. These papular/nodular cancers vary in color, shape, and size, but all such lesions are remarkable for their induration. Secondary changes include thick, hard scale or fissuring with crust. These SCC can erode and even ulcerate, but the keratinization continues to be present. All differentiated SCC occur on sun-exposed areas of skin as UVR is their main etiologic factor. Women commonly develop these skin cancer subtypes on their legs, whereas men display them on their shoulders, back and face.

Invasive SCC can be undifferentiated as well. In which case, the lesion's appearance differs from the above described well differentiated SCC's. Undifferentiated lesions lack keratosis. Thus, they are soft to palpation. The typical lesions range from papules to nodules to "cauliflower-like" vegetations and are usually poorly marginated with extremely friable surfaces. The early lesions will usually erode or ulcerate, but maintain a soft, fleshy border. Poorly differentiated invasive SCC can be singular or multiple and are most commonly seen on the genitalia. Like well differentiated SCC, these invasive forms arise from previous in-situ lesions. Thus, if an undifferentiated lesion is on the genitalia, it probably began as erythroplasia of queyrat, whereas non-genital lesions arise from Bowen's disease.

The appearance of cutaneous SCC is notable different from mucous membrane SCC. Cutaneous SCC are usually displayed on areas of sun exposed skin. Thus, they are most commonly well differentiated and display the typical keratinized, indurated papular/nodular appearance of such SCC. Other dermatoheliosis are commonly displayed concomitantly. The large majority of cutaneous SCC occur on the head and neck regions of the body-accounting for > 75% of all cutaneous SCC.

Mucous membrane SCC differ in appearance from cutaneous forms of the epithelial skin cancer. This variety is usually a moist, velvety, soft erythematous plaque or nodule with possible erosion, ulceration or secondary thickening. The most common site for SCC of mucous membrane origin is the lip—especially the lower lip. These SCC arise from an area of leukoplakia or a previously actinic lesion. These mucous membrane SCC—when invasive may be either well differentiated or poorly differentiated with the later form predominating. A thorough examination of the gross lesion will usually delineate between the two forms. A biopsy should always be performed to confirm your suspicions. Those SCC that originate from mucous membrane are more commonly undifferentiated and thus, are more likely to metastasize to regional nodes and distant locals than cutaneous hyperkeratotic SCC.

DIAGNOSIS AND TREATMENT

The diagnosis and treatment options for SCC are quite similar to BCC. This information was previously outlined in the same section of the BCC portion of this chapter. Please refer to these pages for a description of the diagnosis and treatment of SCC.

MANAGEMENT

To Manage

▼ Keep—any biopsy confirmed SCC that:
   1. Is not a recurrence
   2. Is not in the high-risk facial area
   3. Is not > 2 cm in diameter
   4. Is not a morphea form variant of SCC
▼ Treat:
   1. Small (< 0.5 cm) superficial lesions with cryotherapy or electrodesiccation and curettage.
   2. Large lesions (0.5 cm–2 cm diameter) with elliptical excision and primary closure.

▼ Educate:

1. Importance of follow-up visits and self-examination to monitor any recurrence of a lesion.
2. Liberal use of sunscreen
3. Return between annual check-ups if any new lesions develop
4. High risk factors for developing BCC/SCC discussed

Send

▼ Any biopsy proven SCC that:

1. Is recurrent (to Mohs)
2. Is in the high-risk facial area (to Mohs)
3. Is > 2 cm in diameter (excision with complex closure)
4. Is a morphea form variant (to Mohs)

▼ Any questionable lesion < 0.5 cm in diameter for collaborative opinion.

PROGNOSIS

Although SCC is associated with greater morbidity than BCC, the former has a remission rate of ~90% after proper therapy. The concern with SCC is its ability to metastasize. Thus, early diagnosis of these skin cancers remains key in the overall disease prognosis and cost control. Remember undifferentiated SCC and mucous membrane SCC are at the greatest risk for metastasis

SCC requires close follow-up due to its potential to metastasize. Local recurrence is usually within 2 years of initial therapy whereas metastasis are commonly seen within 5 years. It is best to follow SCC patients every 3 months for the first year after diagnosis/treatment, then every 3–6 months for the next 2 years. For years 4 and 5 the patient can be seen every 6–12 months. If no further abnormality is found at 5 year status-post treatment of SCC, yearly visits are generally sufficient.

PEARLS AND PITFALLS

Risk factors for SCC are listed in Table 7.3.

Perform a thorough history

Attempt to identify all possible etiologic risk factors for each individual patient.

TABLE 7.3 ▼ Predisposing Factors for SCCLD

Sunlight (UVB) exposure	HPV
Artificial light exposure	Oral PUVA
Outdoor occupation	Immunosuppression
Male sex	Arsenic
Fair skin/light eyes and hair	Discoid SLE
Chronic ulcers	Topical nitrogen mustard
Industrial chemicals	Chronic scarring
(Tar, soot, coal, pitch	Burn scars
Fuel oil, creosote)	AIDS, immunosuppression
Sunbather	

Be certain to include examination of regional lymph nodes when discovering a suspicious lesion.

Many SCC are missed at early stages due to their papulosquamous appearance. Fixed papulosquamous lesions (nodules, plaques or ulcers) that persist for one month or more should be evaluated for SCC.

Diagnostic delay can have serious prognostic consequences.

Watch dermatoheliosis, mucous membrane lesions, and genital lesions very closely. Biopsy an abnormal area if *any* question of possible SCC. Consult as needed.

In-situ SCC closely mimics eczema or psoriasis. Especially watch persistent or quick growing/changing lesions. If any question a biopsy should be performed for diagnostic confirmation.

CASE 7.5

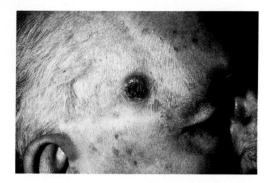

S: A 68-year-old male presents to your clinic for follow-up on his hypertension. He is a retired carpenter who moved to the Miami area 3 months prior to his appointment. He had previously been a lifetime resident of Nashville, Tennessee. He states his only known medical illness is the hypertension. He has history of a T-A as a child and right knee arthroscopy about 10 years prior. Family history is benign. Medications include only 10 mg of Adoral each day.

O: Well-nourished, healthy adult male who appears his stated age. His BP is 134/78 and rest of vitals are stable.

Examination of the skin shows many discrete, brown macular lesions over the forehead, face, and neck. Moderate photoaging is present as well. The right temple displays a well demarcated discrete, erythematous nodule with central ulceration. The surrounding skin is non-affected. No evidence of excoriation or recent trauma. There exists no lymphadenopathy. The rest of his exam, including cardiovascular, is non-remarkable.

NOTE: When questioned about temple lesion the patient states it has been present for 6 months and "doesn't want to heal up."

Tests/Studies: Punch biopsy of right temple nodule shows squamous cell carcinoma.

A: 1. Well controlled hypertension
2. Multiple facial solar lentigo
3. Photoaged skin
4. Squamous cell carcinoma right temple

P: 1. Continue on dose of Aderal. Recheck in 6 months.
2. Stable—No cosmetic treatment desired
3. Stable—No cosmetic treatment desired
4. Referral to dermatologist for full excision and histopathologic examination.

PATIENT EDUCATION HANDOUT
EPITHELIAL SKIN TUMORS

You have been diagnosed with a skin cancer known as: Basal cell carcinoma or Squamous cell carcinoma.

This is not a type of melanoma, but is still a malignant or cancerous growth.

The most common cause of this skin cancer is sunlight or artificial light (as in tanning beds)

Prevention is the key:

> Use sunscreen. At least 15 SPF. Liberally
> Reapply sunscreen if sweating or water exposure
> Use moisturizers with sunscreen
> Wear protective clothing whenever out in the sunlight
> Avoid outdoors from 10 am to 3 pm if possible

There are other causes of skin cancers such as yours. Your doctor will go over these with you to see if you have any of these risk factors. Follow-up visits are very important in keeping your cancer from becoming more serious. *Do not* miss an appointment even if the skin the tumor was taken off or looks "ok."

▶ HELIOSIS

How we look is an important concern for patients today. Plainly the most common cosmetic problem is heliosis. "Heliosis" refers to the group of skin disorders that are induced by exposure to light, especially high energy short-wave length light. A similar and often synonymous term is "photosensitivity." Helioses are numerous and we will discuss the most common of these in this text. The helioses seen most often in primary care setting include: sunburn, photo aging, photosensitivity/photoallergy, solar lentigo, solar (actinic) keratosis, and solar (PMLE) urticaria.

▶ Sunburn

BACKGROUND

Summer sunburn is an acute, common, delayed, transitory and inflammatory skin injury which follows the skin's exposure to ultraviolet light-natural or artificial. Ultraviolet radiation (UVR) consists of UVA and UVB wavelengths. It is the UVB form of ultraviolet light that is 85% responsible for sunburn. During the winter months, when the earths axis is tipped away from the sun, less UVB reaches the surface of the earth and sunburn is rare. Remember, at high altitudes, the atmosphere is thinner and less able to filter out UVB. Thus, sunlight will more produce sunburn in these high regions than at lower altitudes. UVB is not reflected off water and it can penetrate clean clouds. The dose of UVB also depends upon the time of day, latitude, reflection, shade, air contamination, and presence or absence of sunscreens.

Sunburn is most commonly seen in fair skinned individuals. These patients have low amounts of melanin in their epithelial cells. It is this pigment that reduces the ability of light to induce a inflammatory skin reaction. Thus, fair-skinned persons have low amounts of melanin and a reduced ability to absorb electrons or filter out the light and so are more likely to develop sunburn than are darker skinned individuals. But, even those individuals with brown or black skin can develop a sunburn if their exposure to the sunlight is for a long enough duration. Interestingly, young children and elderly adults have a decreased ability to sunburn.

The pathogenesis and etiology of sunburn are still being studied. All the exact molecules or chromophores that absorb the UVB light are not yet known. Prostaglandins produce most of the sunburn reaction. It is generally felt that DNA defects play an important role in UVB induced epithelial injury both immediate and long-term.. Exposure to UVB light will lead to microscopic changes in various epidermal cells within 30 minutes of the actual exposure. These changes involve exocytosis of leukocytes, and vacuolization of melanocytes and Langerhans cells. UVB light-affectation of these various intra-epidermal elements triggers the release of certain mediators which include prostaglandin, lysosomal enzymes, cytokines, serotonin and kinins. It is the release of these intracellular mediators which induces the endothelial cell edema and dermal erythema characteristic of sunburn.

IN THE CLINIC

The clinical appearance of sunburn will vary based on its severity. Most sunburn is characterized by a macular pink to red confluent erythema and mild to moderate edema well-demarcated from sun-protected skin. Under the microscope, we find microvesicles. Those areas of severe sunburn demonstrate intense erythema, moderate to severe edema, crusts, and blistering. These patients appear quite ill with possible constitutional symptoms including fever, chills, malaise, headache and nausea. Mild sunburn is typically pruritic while severe vesicular sunburn is intensely painful.

The above clinical signs and symptoms of sunburn will initially appear approximately 4–6 hours after sun exposure and then peak at 12–24 hours. If the patient remains out of the UVR exposure after a sunburn, all of the clinical findings should fade within 3–5 days.

DIAGNOSIS AND MANAGEMENT

The diagnosis of sunburn is purely clinical. Photosensitivity reactions can closely mimic sunburn. Consider a photo sensitivity reaction if: 1) the burn is immediate; 2) the burn is too severe for the dose of sunlight; 3) the burn includes urticaria or papules [not seen in sunburn]; 4) the burn persists after 96 hours (4 days); and 5) the sunburn produces an unnatural pattern on the skin.

The treatment of sunburn varies with the severity of the disease. Mild reactions are treated topically with cool-water wet dressings or baths every 4–6 hours along with mid-potency corticosteroids twice each day. Fifty-percent dilution of the topical steroid ointment with cold ice water allows for easier application of the medium to the painful surface of the skin. Oral treatment of mild sunburn includes acetylsalicylic acid for pain and antihistamines for any associated pruritus. Numerous studies have been performed on the use of NSAID's for sunburn analgesia and the results are mixed. Those studies that have found these medications to be helpful have advocated giving the doses of specific NSAID as early in the course of the disease process as possible.

Severe sunburn needs the same topical treatment as more mild reactions. Oral analgesia with and NSAID or acetylsalicylic acid is often moderately helpful. Since pruritus is rarely a symptom, and the process is not histamine mediated, antihistamines is rarely of any benefit. A short 7 day oral corticosteroid taper may be initiated in these patients, but, use of systemic corticosteroids in severe sunburn is purely anecdotal and all controlled studies up to date have not shown this treatment to be efficacious. Bed rest and basic burn dressing is advised for those severe sunburn patients whose reactions include constitutional symptoms.

The best method of managing sunburn is via prevention. Proper clothing, shelter, avoiding exposure to sunlight from 10am to 3pm, tanning bed abstinence, and judicious use of sunscreens with an SPF of 15 or greater are all methods by which sunburn can be prevented.

MANAGEMENT

To Manage

▼ Keep all cases
▼ Treat—topically
▼ Cool water compresses for 15–20 minutes every 4–6 hours.
▼ Cool water baths every 4–6 hours
▼ Mid potency corticosteroid cream/ointment twice each day
  Systemically
  Acetylsalicylic acid PRN pain
  Mild sunburn—antihistamines every 8 hours PRN pruritus
  Severe sunburn—Corticosteroid taper over 7 days.
▼ Prevention/Patient Education
  Proper clothing, hats, sunglasses

Sunscreen use—SPF 15 or greater; zinc oxide ointment

Avoid sunlight from 10 am–3 pm,

Do not use tanning beds

PROGNOSIS

Most sunburn heals fully without any subsequent scar formation. A few cases of this common heliosis will lead to permanent hypopigmentation which is most likely related to melanocyte destruction. Also, repeated sunburn in patients will eventually lead to photo aging overtime. A history of multiple severe, blistering sunburn as a child is a known risk factor for epidermal malignant melanoma as an adult.

PEARLS AND PITFALLS

▼ Systemic lupus erythematosus SLE can cause an erythema that often mimics sunburn. Photo allergy looks like allergic contact dermatitis.

▼ Sunburn cannot be classified according to depth as 1st degree, 2nd degree, or 3rd degree.

▼ Topical anesthetics are not effective at treatment of sunburn, and can in fact, potentially sensitize the skin.

▼ These lubricants which contain significant amounts of fragrance can sensitize the skin to sunburn and irritate skin that is suffering from this form of heliosis.

▼ Sunburns can trigger other diseases such as pustular psoriasis, porphyria or herpes simplex, that are not helioses. The cause of these diseases is simply the injury to skin induced by the sunburn.

▶ PHOTOAGING

BACKGROUND

Photo aging, also known as dermatoheliosis, develops as a result of repeated and prolonged exposure to UVR from the sun or from artificial tanning beds. This photo damage of the epidermis begins when the patient is young and is compounded as the same individuals re-expose their skin to UVR repeatedly as they age. The degree of photo aging of the skin is dependent upon various factors. These factors include the patient's skin color and ability to tan as well as the time exposed to UVR and the light's actual intensity.

The individuals most likely to develop early photo aging are those fair skinned people who tan poorly and burn easily. Although possible, this type of heliosis is almost never observed in those patients who are black or dark-brown in skin color. The skin changes are usually not manifested until at least the fourth decade of life and are more common in men than women. The development of this form of heliosis is more likely in those patients who inhabit climates where the intensity of UVR is severe-such as the southern coast or at high altitudes, and especially, if these same people are out in the sunlight for long periods of time as a child, teen, and/or young adult. Patients such as life guards and farmers whose profession requires such long-time exposure to UVR are especially at risk for suffering from dermatoheliosis in early adulthood.

The development of photoaged skin occurs slowly over time. The exposure of susceptible epidermis to UVR-especially UVB-leads to concomitant cellular atypia and acanthosis. The deeper skin layers experience an increase in elastosis, and collagen. Some basic science studies have shown UVA light to cause similar skin changes in mice. But, no studies to date have demonstrated UVA as a definitive etiology of photoaging in humans.

IN THE CLINIC

The patient with photoaged skin appears much older than their actual chronologic age. These people not only have extremely xerotic skin but also manifest other skin changes as outlined in Table 7.4. These skin changes can be manifested on any epidermis often exposed to UVR. Commonly affected skin includes that covering the shoulders, back, chest, face, scalp and upper extremities.

DIAGNOSIS AND TREATMENT

Diagnosis of photo aging is clinical-based on both history and physical findings. Rarely is further investigation necessary. Treatment of photoaged skin is quite limited. Topical tretinoin (ex. Retin-A, Differin, Azelex acid, Renova) has been proven in various controlled clinical trials to be moderately effective in the treatment of dermatoheliosis. These medications actually reverse some of the photo damaged induced earlier in life. Chemical peeling is an option, but ex-

TABLE 7.4 ▼ Skin Manifestations of
Photo Aging

Xerosis
Solar keratosis
Solar lentigo
Telangiectasias
Wrinkling
Freckles
Purpura
Elastosis
Yellowing
Atrophy
Easy bruising
Skin cancer

pense, recovery time, and mismatch with "unpeeled" skin are all limitations. Laser therapy is gaining in popularity. Although quite economically burdensome, the results of this mode of treatment are quite positive. Unfortunately, as with all newer therapy modalities, the long-term results are not yet known.

The key to treatment of all photo aging is prevention. Those fair-skinned patients who burn easily and tan rarely should be warned about the effects the sun or UV tanning beds can have on their skin in time. The same prevention rules apply to dermatoheliosis as to sunburn: Use of sunscreens, avoiding peak hours of sunlight, proper clothing. Also, those at risk patients should be taught to never "sunbathe" and should be prudent about using such protective lubricants on skin everyday.

MANAGEMENT

To Manage

▼ Keep all cases of photo aging.

▼ Treatment

▼ Topical tretinoin preparation of your choice once daily. (Follow guidelines as specific for each type.) Allow 6–8 weeks for beginning improvement.

▼ If this topical treatment fails—Consult dermatologist—for possible referral as below.

▼ Biopsy any possible melanoma, basal cell carcinomas.

Send

For consult on chemical peel/laser treatment

PROGNOSIS

If dermatoheliosis is left untreated its course is progressive. Even if the patient develops judicious sun exposure practices later in life, the damage wrought at an early age will continue to manifest itself over time. The various treatment options outlined above may aid in reversal of the dermatoheliosis, but the patient must be vigilant about avoiding prolonged or frequent UVR exposure without protection in the future.

PEARLS AND PITFALLS

- ▼ Prevention is the key to managing photoaging, and epithelial skin cancer.
- ▼ Attempt to incorporate patient education on photoaging into your health maintenance examinations.
- ▼ Posters/pictures of wrinkled, wrened, photoaged skin often make an impact on the patients perceptions of a "healthy tan."
- ▼ All the currently available treatment options are expensive and not reimbursed by insurance companies.

▶ PHOTOSENSITIVITY

BACKGROUND

In this text we will review only the most common etiology of photosensitivity—that which is drug induced. Drugs need not be systemically dosed to cause a photosensitive reaction. Topical application of various medications can lead to photosensitivity as easily as do some ingested medications. When certain drugs are used simultaneously with exposure to sun or UVR the characteristic skin changes can be seen. The drugs that in combination with light can lead to photosensitivity reactions are listed in Table 7.5.

Photo toxicity and photo allergy are the two forms of drug-induced photosensitivity. These heliosis can occur in any race, ethnicity, sex, or age group, although photoallergy is more common in the adult population. The reason for an increased incidence of photoal-

TABLE 7.5 ▼ Drugs That Can Cause Photosensitivity Reactions

Photo allergic	Photo toxic
Benzocaine	Amiodarone
Benzophenone	Coal tar
Neomycin	Dilantin
PABA	Doxycycline
Perfumes/fragrances	Furosemide (limes, lemons,
Phenothiazine	carrots, celery)
Quinidine	Griseofulvin
Quinine	Halidixic acid
Retinoids	Naliclixic acid
Salicylanilide	NSAIDs
6 methylcoumcum	Piroxicam
(sunscreen)	Psoralens (plants)
Stilbene (whitener)	Sulfonamides
Sulfonamides	
Tetracycline	
Thiazides	

lergy with age is thought to be a result of it's delayed hypersensitivity mechanism of occurrence. Like all Type IV allergic reactions—delayed hypersensitivity to a drug requires an initial exposure to the same agent at an earlier age in order to "sensitize" the individual. Photoallergy requires the drug to be present in the skin. When simultaneously exposed to UVR, the drug and light combine to form a "photo-drug." This entity precedes to bind with proteins to form an antigen. Antibodies to this antigen are formed via the immune system. Thus, the next occasion the same drug is taken simultaneous to light exposure and the same photo-drug product is formed if it is attacked by the preformed antibodies and a photo allergic response is born. Unlike photoallergy, phototoxity does not involve the immune system and is rather a more direct epidermal response to simultaneous drug and light exposure.

Rather than inducing the formation of a "photo-drug" antigen, the UVR/drug exposure causes certain toxic free radicals to be released in the epidermis and underlying dermis. These free radicals attack the cellular structures of the skin and lead to the typical cutaneous changes of photo toxicity.

Interestingly UVA light, which is responsible for only a small portion of sunburn, is the type of UVR that induces photo dermatosis. It is UVA that is relatively plentiful in the winter months and often photo dermatosis occurs during outdoor activities such as skiing and ice skating.

IN THE CLINIC

Acute **photo allergic** skin reactions closely resemble a severe, acute, contact dermatitis (Chapter 7.1) The cutaneous changes are eczematous with poor margination, mild to moderate erythema, and a degree of vesiculation, weeping, and crust formation dependent on the degree of hypersensitivity the patient has developed. The rash usually involves those areas of skin which were uncovered at the time of insult, but the neighboring, protected epidermis may demonstrate similar changes. If the cutaneous photo allergic response is not treated it will change over time and appear more like a chronic irritant contact dermatitis. These alterations are due to the pruritic nature of all photoallergy. The patient responds to the itch by scratching the affected skin. Over time, this repetitive cutaneous trauma will cause lichenification, excoriation, and scaling. These disorders may last for years.

   Photo toxicity presents clinically quite differently than its eczema-like photo allergic cousin. Within 2–4 hours the patients skin develops a mild, red appearance. At about 12 hours, the cutaneous changes of this photo dermatitis include *intense* erythema and edema with significant degrees of vesiculation bulla formation and subsequent weeping and crusting. The underlying bright red alterations appear clinically much like a severe sunburn. But, the secondary vesiculation is more pronounced than would be expected for the duration of time the patient is typically exposed to the insulting light. Unlike photoallergy, this "exaggerated sunburn" is seen *only* on those portions of a patient's skin that was exposed to the UVA light. Nails may be involved if psoralens or tetracycline is the culprit medication. Nail changes with these photo toxic drugs are limited to photo-onycholysis.

DIAGNOSIS AND TREATMENT

The diagnosis of both forms of photo dermatosis is usually clinical. Obtaining a thorough history-including medications and light exposure—is critical to determining the offending drug. Remember, skin changes that resemble a terrible sunburn, severe, confluent edema and erythema with overlying vesicles and bulla are due to a drug induced Photo toxic reaction. Photoallergy induces an eczematous rash that appears much like a "poison ivy" dermatitis induced by smoke from the burning of wood covered with this plant or its resin. Photo testing for the responsible pharmaceutical/plant is more likely to be necessary in photoallergy reaction than in Photo toxic drug reactions. Elderly patients or others who are using multiple possible etiologic drugs may need this special testing to determine which drug is the inciting agent. Photo testing is quite complex and is best performed by a dermatologist familiar with its intricacies.

Drug-induced dermatoheliosis are treated with removal of the offending drug and staying out of UVR as much as possible until the skin manifestations resolve. The patient should be warned about future use of the responsible drug. Otherwise, the patient should be treated symptomatically with cool water compresses/soaks, topical mid-potency corticosteroids twice-a-day and systemic antihistamines every 8 hours to relieve the pruritus. If the photo dermatosis is severe, a short (7–10 day) taper of oral corticosteroids may be beneficial.

MANAGEMENT

To Manage

▼ Keep all cases initially

▼ Remove the patient from UV light. Cover up.

▼ Treat—*Mostly topicals only*

▼ Topical cold water compresses/baths every 4 hours to help relieve pruritus.

▼ Topical mid-potency corticosteroid twice a day

▼ Oral antihistamine every 8 hours as needed for pruritus

▼ *If severe*—systemic corticosteroid taper over 7–10 days

▼ Patient education:

Determine drug responsible and stop this medication

Warn about future use of the specific drug

Send

Any photo dermatitis where responsible drug not easily determined or initial history/examination or persists despite removal of likely etiologic agent.

To dermatologist for photo patch testing.

PROGNOSIS

All photo toxic drug reactions by definition will resolve when the responsible substance is stopped. The majority of photo allergic drug rashes remit under the same conditions. The recovery may be prolonged. Some photo allergic cutaneous changes can continue for weeks to years despite removal of the causative drug from the patients environment. Such persistent photoallergy can be quite emotionally disabling to the patient and the physician should be appropriately sympathetic. Avoidance of all UV light may be required for several months, systemic steroids may be needed, and the process is tedious.

PEARLS AND PITFALLS

▼ In photo allergic drug reactions it is more difficult to determine the etiologic medication. These cases more commonly need referral than drug induced photo toxic rashes. Collaborate with your dermatologist.

▼ Patient education important in preventing a recurrence.

▼ Use systemic corticosteroids:
  1. Rarely
  2. Only if symptoms are severe
  3. Never as a substitute for prompt etiologic diagnosis
  4. Never long term for persistent photoallergy.

▼ Be thorough in your history taking. If you have a doubt over drug responsible—send for photo patch testing.

Solar Urticaria

The topic of artificial UVR or sun-induced urticarial reactions was fully discussed in Chapter 7. Please refer to this chapter for further discussion of this form of heliosis. A mixed photo-induced rash called polymorphous light eruption is partly papules, part vesicles and part urticaria. It is seen early in the spring and responds well to topical steroids. This is most common type of photo urticaria.

Solar Lentigo (Not Lentigo Maligna)

These discrete macular areas of epidermal hyper pigmentation will be mentioned only briefly in this text. Solar lentigo develop in light-skinned individuals who have been exposed to sunlight or artificial UVR for a substantial period of time throughout their lives. They develop due to localized UVR induced melanocyte proliferation. These :sun-spots: are usually initially manifested around 40 year olds and are more common in those who have spent a portion of their lifetime in warm, southern climates. Solar lentigo are never seen in dark-skinned or black populations, but can occur in Asian individuals.

All solar lentigo are macular without any palpable substance by definition. They are usually oval or round, range in size from 1.0–4.0 cm in diameter, and increase in size slowly. Their dark to light brown hyperpigmentation allows for easy demarcation from the surrounding skin. The lesions can be seen on any area of epidermis that has experienced chronic sun exposure.

Treatment of solar lentigo can be cost-effectively carried out in the primary care clinic. Topic tretinoin and azelaic acid applied once daily can often lighten these hyper pigmented macules enough to allow them to become indistinguishable from the surrounding skin. A single episode of Cryotherapy for 10 seconds is an effective therapy as well. Those solar lentigo that are unresponsive to the above modalities or are large (4–5 cm in diameter) are best treated with laser therapy. Unfortunately, this mode of therapy is costly and is not reimbursable by insurance companies for such "cosmetic" uses.

Chemical peels are also a referral option. The patient with solar lentigo is likely to have other skin manifestations of chronic UVR exposure. Thus, chemical peeling is an option to treat the entire affected area. Like lasers, this cosmetic treatment option is expensive and should only be performed by experienced dermatologist or plastic surgeons. Be wary of the cosmetologist who offers chemical peels. In unexperienced hands this treatment can be highly dangerous and could result in permanently damaged skin.

Solar (Actinic) Keratosis

This type of heliosis is discussed at length in Chapter 8. (Epithelial skin cancer). Only 1 squamous cell cancer will develop per 1000 actinic keratosis each year. But, the general population has been sensitized to see these lesions as "precancers" and often present to the primary care clinic for their removal. Please refer to Chapter 9.6 for further discussion of these scaly forms of heliosis.

CASE 7.6

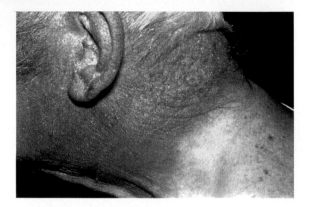

S: A 44-year-old executive from Arlington, Virginia is alarmed about a painful persisting sunburn. Last Friday afternoon he played 18 holes of golf, and noticed a sunburn that evening although he had a tan, and hadn't burned on prior outings. On Sunday, he was still burned and his wife became concerned. He actually felt worse on Monday morning when he talked his way past your nurse and into your clinic on Washington Circle. He has had recurring acne rosacea for some years, and is currently taking tetracycline 250 mg TID, but otherwise no medications. He claims to be entirely healthy.

O: A slightly overweight, well-groomed man looks older than 42 years old. He is afebrile, has normal vital signs and complains of nothing other than his skin. Strikingly over his face, neck, ears, hands, and arms to-the-sleeve, he has an even red dermatitis with spots of crusting, looking just like a sunburn.

A: Phototoxic eczematoid dermatitis, very likely due to tetracycline.

P: Strict avoidance of all outdoor light is necessary for a few days. Use hat, sleeves and gloves. Protect the skin on cloudy days. Cool wet dressings 30 minutes every hour, as possible, for 48 hours will give relief. A triamcinolone cream may be used. List the case as an adverse drug reaction. The patient may have to avoid the sun for some weeks or even months, and miss out on his golf.

PATIENT EDUCATION HANDOUT

HELIOSIS

Your physician has diagnosed you with a skin disease called_____. This disease was due to damage from light over exposure.

You have been prescribed a medication called_____.
Directions to use include:_____

If you have sunburn or sun/drug rash you may also:
>—Place cool water soaks or take cool water baths every 4–6 hours
>—OTC or prescribed antihistamines:_____
>To help with itching
>—Aspirin—2 tabs every 4–6 hours for pain.

If you have been told to stop taking a medication be certain to do so.

If you have photo damaged skin, realize that unprotected exposure to the sun in the future will worsen the changes, but, remaining out of the sun does not mean your skin damage will not worsen.

The photo damage you see today is from the sun you received many years ago.

A dermatologist can treat some photo aging with lasers or chemical peels. These are *not covered by insurance* and can be expensive. If you are interested, ask your doctor.

Call with any questions/concerns.

▶ PALPABLE PURPURA

BACKGROUND

Palpable purpura are those skin lesions classically associated with vasculitis. But, the clinically awkward concept of vasculitis makes the classification of palpable purpura quite difficult to explain and to utilize in the clinic.

Vasculitis is the term employed to describe a set of clinical disorders defined by typical histological abnormalities within blood vessels (see Table 7.6). These microscopic changes include segmental inflammation of blood vessel walls with accompanying inflammatory cellular infiltrates and fibrin deposits. The type of vasculitis seen clinically depends upon the size and location of the involved blood vessels.

The vasculitides that demonstrate palpable purpura involve small cutaneous blood vessels, usually the post-capillary venules. These venules are the vessels primarily affected in patients with cutaneous, or hypersensitivity vasculitis. Thus, palpable purpura are the classic lesions seen in cutaneous vasculitis (Table 7.7) best exemplified by drug reactions. But, small-vessel skin changes are also seen in other vasculitides such as Wegener's granulomatosis, temporal arteritis (TA) and polyarteritis nodosa (PAN). Thus, these vasculitides which primarily involve other, non-cutaneous vessels, may demonstrate palpable purpura in addition to other clinical manifestations. Infrequently, diseases other than pure vasculitis can cause palpable purpura. Such disorders include Dengue fever, trauma, orthostasis, subacute bacterial endocarditis, disseminated intravascular coagulation, and Sweets syndrome. These diseases will not be covered in our text.

To further confuse the issue, cutaneous vasculitis may have systemic involvement as well as the purpuric rash. The organs typically affected are the kidney, liver, and GI tract. Cutaneous vasculitis in

---

TABLE 7.6 ▼ Causes of Palpable Purpura

Cutaneous vasculitis (Table 7.7)	Rocky Mountain spotted fever
Subacute bacterial endocarditis	Amyloidosis
Trauma	Disseminated intravascular
Bacteremia	coagulation
Sweet's Syndrome	Amyloidosis

TABLE 7.7 ▼ Cutaneous Vasculitis

Idiopathic Neoplasms	
—Nodular vasculitis	Connective Tissue Disease
—Wenloch-Schonlein purpura	Rheumatoid Arthritis
Recurrent urticarial syndrome	SLE
Livedoid vasculitis	Sjogren's Syndrome
Acute hemorrhagic edema	Raynaud Disease
of childhood	Cryoglobinemia
Infectious disease	
Bacterial paraproteinemia	
Viral ulcerative colitis	
Cystic fibrosis	
Serum Sickness Drug Induced	
Penicillin	
Sulfonamides	
Thiazides	
NSAIDs	
Allopurinol	
Phenytoin	

the adult is most commonly due to an idiopathic etiology with drug-induced causes running a close second. But, cutaneous vasculitis and its associated palpable purpura may also result from various infections, collagen vascular diseases, neoplasms, embolic phenomena and other chronic diseases (Table 7.7).

The exact pathologic mechanism behind the histologic changes seen with palpable purpura is not fully known. As with all the clinical findings of the vasculitides, circulating immune complexes are thought to play a role. The exact type of vasculitis and its corresponding clinical presentation depend upon which blood vessels these immune complexes deposit themselves into. One deposited, the immune complex will activate the complement cascade either directly or via interaction with cell membrane receptors. Either way, the number of neutrophils and other anaphylatoxins present locally

TABLE 7.8 ▼ Vasculitis

Temporal arteritis	Polyarteritis nodosa
Churgg Strauss arteritis	CNS vasculitis
Wegeners granulomatosis	Connective tissue diseases
Hypersensitivity vasculitis	

radically increases. The cellular infiltrates eventually lead to necrosis of the involved vascular segment and the formation of fibrin deposits. In cutaneous vasculitis the blood vessels affected are the venules. The vascular permeability and cellular infiltrate composition leads to the formation of the palpable purpura seen on clinical examination.

IN THE CLINIC

What exactly do we mean by essential palpable purpura? *Essential* refers to a absence of other concomitant *skin* diseases. Such as herpes simplex, bug bites, eczema. These cutaneous disorders can present with secondary purpura—usually as a result of picking or scratching. *Purpura* are erythematous lesions that are non-blanchable unlike telangiectasias. This inability to blanch is best demonstrated via pressing a clear slide against the lesion and watching for a disappearance of color. Purpura can be further subdivided by size into petechiae (<3 mm diameter) and ecchymosis (> 3 cm diameter). If a significant amount of edema is associated with a lesion it is known as contusion. *Palpable* purpura are those non-blanchable erythematous lesions that are raised. Thus, palpable purpura are papular and not macular in their basic morphology. The majority of non-palpable purpura are a result of intravascular abnormality—notably platelet defects or coagulopathies. Thus, a good physical examination of the suspect rash must be performed. The examinations need to include palpation of the lesions. If the skin is not touched, the examiner cannot determine if a lesion is palpable or even whether or not it is purpuric.

The palpable purpura of cutaneous vasculitis is usually found on localized areas of the lower extremities. The lesions are usually small and they vary in shape from round to annular. They may be discrete or confluent and remain stable in size. The lesions may be asymptomatic or they may be pruritic, burning or painful. The purpura last days to weeks without change in shape or size until they fade. Lesions may be recurrent over a period of years with new ones arising as the old ones fade. The palpable purpura characteristic of a cutaneous vasculitude may present with other primary lesions. These basic lesions will vary depending on which vasculitis is involved. Some examples are nodules (PAN, TA), ulcers, pustules, and vesicles. The purpuric lesions are usually quite violaceous at their borders with the nodules, ulcers, etc . . . arising towards the center of the erythematous skin change. Wheals may occur in urticarial forms of vasculitis.

Palpable purpura may be the primary manifestation of the vasculitis. This scenario is what is demonstrated in the hypersensitivity vasculitudes (Table 7.8). Whether the skin is the predominant organ effected by the vasculitis or not, the possibility of systemic involvement should always be investigated. Organs commonly effected include the CNS, peripheral nerves, kidney, and the GI tract. Again, do not forget to investigate for underlying disease or organ involvement during your work-up of a patient with palpable purpura.

DIAGNOSIS AND TREATMENT

The clinical challenge when approaching a patient with palpable purpura is to determine if the rash is the result of vasculitis or another disease (Table 7.6). A complete history and physical is vital in establishing a diagnosis.

Question the patient about recent drug ingestion or infection. Ask about sexual history (HIV) and recent camping (Rocky Mountain Spotted fever). Recent weight loss or other signs and symptoms of possible neoplasm. Symptoms of Raynaud phenomena, pleurisy, arthralgias increase the likelihood of possible connective tissue disorder. A history of upper respiratory symptoms or productive cough are associated with Wegener Granulomatosis. A child with palpable purpura, gastrointestinal symptoms, and melanotic stools is likely to be afflicted with Henoch-Schonlein purpura.

If you suspect drug ingestion as the etiology of the purpura the drug should be stopped. This discontinuation of the inciting agent will thus provide both a treatment and an etiologic diagnosis. If the patient has a history of ulcerative colitis, cystic fibrosis, or connective tissue disorder the purpura is most likely a result of the chronic underlying disease. The palpable purpura will improve once therapy specific for the underlying disease is initiated.

Unless clinical examination demonstrates a clear diagnosis, laboratory evaluation is necessary to determine the etiology of the palpable purpura. Start with a sedimentation rate, complete blood count with differential, antinuclear antibody serum complement level, serum rheumatoid factor, urinalysis, blood urea nitrogen, and liver enzymes. Choose these tests coinciding with your clinical suspicion. These basic laboratory values will often aid in establishing a diagnosis. A biopsy of the cutaneous lesions may prove helpful if your diagnosis remains unclear after clinical and laboratory evaluation. A biopsy aids in distinguishing the non-vasculitis causes of palpable purpura. Unfortunately, the histopathological changes seen on skin biopsy of the vasculitides are often similar. Thus, biopsy does not prove fruitful in these cases. Also, bacteremia and Rocky Mountain Spotted Fever have microscopic finding that are often indistinguishable from vasculitis. Be certain to have the dermatologist review the case and the histopathology.

If a full history and physical, laboratory work-up and collaborative biopsy prove unfruitful, the patient should be referred to a dermatologist to confirm your approach and continue the investigation.

The treatment of palpable purpura is based on its etiology. The majority of palpable purpura is due to cutaneous vasculitis. And, most cutaneous vasculitis is idiopathic and self limited. Thus, the majority of palpable purpura is self limited and close over sation is usually all that is warranted. If a drug-induced or infectious purpura is suspected, the rash should resolve after the medication is discontinued or the infection treated. If a chronic disease is the etiology, the purpura will improve once disease—specific therapy is initiated. If a purpuric rash does not spontaneously resolve, is recurrent, or several treatment may be initiated.

In general, all the vasculitides may be treated as follows. Start with oral antihistamines every 6–8 hours in combination with a NSAID every 6–8 hours. Other options in place of or in addition to these agents include hydroxychloroquine sulfate 200 mg a day or colchine 0.6 mg three times each day. If the above does not suffice, it is best to refer or consult a dermatologist. The specialist may then confirm your diagnosis and may decide to initiate higher-risk therapy with oral corticosteroids, immunosuppressive agents or plasmapheresis. The efficaciousness of all the noted therapeutic agents is anecdotal and their use is not based on clinical trial. Follow up with care.

MANAGEMENT

To Manage

▾ Keep all cases initially

▾ Seek etiology—biopsy if necessary with collaboration

▾ Review with your dermatologist any biopsies sent to pathology

▾ Most cutaneous, idiopathic forms are self-limited, not scarring.

▾ If a drug induced etiology—D/C drug immediately

▼ Treat any concomitant infections

▼ Treatment

Oral antihistamines every 6–8 hours with a NSAID every 6–8 hours

Substitute/add: hydroxychloroquinine sulfate 200 mg po every D or

Colchicine 0.6 mg TID

If 1,2,3 fail—Refer to dermatologist

Send

To dermatologist if above treatments fail or if disease state worsens.

PEARLS AND PITFALLS

▼ Periarteritis nodosum is a dangerous vasculitis. The disease is rare. The rash consists of deeply palpable purpura and areas of reticulate necrosis on the legs.

▼ Temporal arteritis is also a rare and dangerous vasculitis. Linear nodules and typical deep palpable painful purpura are demonstrated along the course of an artery. They are often seen on the scalp. These changes lead to alopecia and resultant scalp ulcerations.

▼ Raynaud's Syndrome is also a form of vasculitis. This syndrome recurring digital ischemia occurs in response to cold or mental excitement. The result is pain, numbness, and loss of function. It is sometimes associated with SLE or scleroderma. If Raynaud's is present, persistent or progressive the patient should be worked up for collagen vascular disease.

CASE 7.7

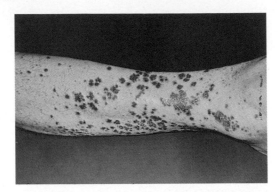

S: A 46-year-old white male presents to your clinic with a rash of 1 weeks duration over his legs that seems to be "spreading" according to the patient. He states the rash is only on his legs and he has never had skin changes like this in the past. The lesions do have associated "burning pain" which has been present since the onset of the eruption. He sates he is otherwise quite healthy and visits a physician only for acute medical problems such as the sore throat he had the week prior which was told was "strep throat" after the doctor swabbed his throat. He is on his 7th day of penicillin and has been feeling much better the last 4 days. He denies any other medical illnesses and is on no other medications. He states he currently feels fine except for the rash and it's associated burning pain.

O: A well nourished, well fed white male who appears his stated age. His vital signs are stable and he is afebrile. The skin over his lower extremities demonstrates multiple, discrete and a few confluent, well-circumscribed purpuric lesions. The lesions are palpably raised and nontender. Pressing a clear glass slide against the lesions shows them to be non-blanchable. The rest of the skin is without abnormality as is the remainder of the physical examination.

A: Palpable purpura. The unremarkable physical examination and patient history point to two possible etiologies. Either the Streptococcus infection itself or the penicillin used to treat the disease.

P: Treat the underlying abnormality. In this case stop the penicillin and replace it with another antibiotic against the streptococcal infection. Follow closely for resolution over the course of a few days to a week. If any further symptoms develop and the rash persists another etiology must be sought.

PATIENT EDUCATION HANDOUT
PALPABLE PURPURA

Your doctor has diagnosed you with a skin disease that has a funny name—"palpable purpura."

There are many things that cause this rash you have and your doctor will talk with you about what might be the reason why you have your rash.

Your doctor has asked you to take the following medications—take only the ones with the box that is checked in front of them.

❏ Benedryl is available over the counter at most grocery stores and pharmacies. It is also called Diphenhydramine. We use this medicine to help with the swelling and the itching of your rash. It is available in a liquid or in a pill form. Your doctor reccommends you take the following dose

_____

❏ Hydrochoroquinine sulfate 200mg—take one tablet one time each day

❏ Colchicine 0.6mg—take one tablet three times a day about eight hours apart

❏ _____

▶ TICK-RELATED DISEASE

The bite of a tick is almost always innocuous. Often times an annular plaque of self-limited erythema, edema and mild pruritus or pain will result. These lesions are best treated with proper wound care to prevent secondary pyoderma. Scarring is rare.

Disease spread by ticks can be quite serious. Unfortunately, the media has dramatized tick bites—especially their potential for transmission of tick borne illness. Many patients will phone or present to your clinic with concern over the possibility of tick borne illness from one tick bite. Due to this fact and due to the serious potential of a tick borne illness, a few diseases deserve mention. This text will focus on Lyme Borreliosis and Rocky Mountain Spotted fever. Although uncommon, these arthropod borne diseases can be fatal if not diagnosed early and managed correctly.

▶ LYME BORRELIOSIS

BACKGROUND

Lyme borreliosis is a multistage tick-borne infectious disease. The spirochete responsible, Borellis burgdorferi is transmitted to humans via the bite of an infected tick. In the U.S. the responsible vector tick is Ixodes—commonly referred to as the deer tick. Ixodes must be attached to human skin for at least 24 hours for transmission of the spirochete. Prompt removal can prevent disease.

Although cases of Lyme Borreliosis have been reported in all 50 states, the multi system disease is most concentrated in the Northeast (May–September) and Pacific Northwest (January–May). The number of cases of Lyme Borreliosis is growing steadily each year as more patients acquire the disease in previously non-indigenous areas. In many states, the ticks do not transmit the disease at all.

IN THE CLINIC

Lyme Borreliosis can be clinically staged into 3 groups based on time from the inciting tick bite (Table 7.9). The first stage occurs from three days to one month after the injury and is typically known as Lyme Disease. The second stage occurs weeks to months after the patient was bitten and involves hematologic dissemination to organ systems. The third stage does not appear for at least one year after the original Ixodes insult. Less than 20% of patients actually recall even being bitten by the vector tick.

Three-fourths of Lyme Borreliosis patients present clinically during the first stage, ie. with typical Lyme Disease. Lyme Disease commonly occurs with an initial rash known as erythema migrans (EM). Erythema migrans is characteristic of Lyme Borreliosis, but is not pathognomic. EM occurs also with the bites of sterile ticks, and with other kinds of bites or stings. EM can be seen in two forms—primary and secondary. Primary EM occurs early in the first stage and rarely has any constitutional symptoms. Whereas secondary EM, which is seen later in the first stage, has predominantly vague systemic complaints.

Primary EM originates at the site of the infected Ixodes bite. At a time when the original punctate wound may no longer visible clinically. A small, erythematous papule arises at the aforementioned cutaneous location. This papular lesion enlarges circumferentially

TABLE 7.9 ▼ Classification of Lyme Borreliosis

Stagetime from Injury	Clinical Finding
I 3 days to 4 weeks	Erythema migrans (Lyme Disease) Primary No constitutional symptoms Secondary Fever, malaise, myalgia, arthralgies
II 3 weeks to months	Arthralgia CNS Possible B. lymphocytoma Cranial neuropathy(s) Meningitis radiculopathim motor/sensory Cardiovascular Myopericarditis AV block LV dysfunction
III 1 year or less	Arthritis mono/periarticular Encephalopathy Acrodermatitis chronica Atrophicus

within days to form a round to oval shaped, florid red to violet colored area of poorly demarcated solid erythema. As this discrete lesion enlarges, it begins to demonstrate rings of shaded erythema. The brightest colors are those at the lesions margins with gradual duskiness and fading towards the center. Primary EM ranges in size from 3 cm to greater than 20 cm in diameter. The annular characteristic predominates as the lesion size increases.

The lesion is typically mildly pruritic but otherwise asymptomatic. The typical skin lesion of primary EM can demonstrate secondary changes such as centralized vesiculation, induration of necrosis. These findings are usually seen in the patient who has a hypersensitivity to tick bites. As previously noted, primary EM is demonstrated where the original tick bite occurred. Thus, it is distributed most commonly in those areas of skin most often bitten by this vector. Such sites include the trunk, axilla, inguinal region, and the proximal extremities.

Secondary EM is seen weeks after the original tick bite. These later skin lesions are multiple in number and are displayed in crops at sites distant from the primary EM. This may be discrete but often overlap. Otherwise, the clinical appearance of each separate secondary EM is similar to primary EM as noted above. By the time these secondary lesions occur, the primary lesion is usually fully resolved.

Secondary EM is notable for its significant constitutional symptoms. Patient often complain of headache, myalgia, low grade fever, malaise, arthralgia. At times these symptoms are quite severe and may be patients presenting complaint.

A less common skin manifestation of Lyme disease is known as lymphocytoma cutis or Borrelia Lymphocytoma. This discrete solitary nodule usually presents later in the first stage of Lyme Borreliosis (i.e. Lyme Disease) when secondary EM is manifested. The 3 cm to 5 cm diameter nodule red to brown in color, asymptomatic, and distributed on the head, nipples, scrotum, axilla, or extremities. The earlobe is the most common site for this persistent nodule.

The second and third stages of Lyme Borreliosis are clinically characterized by disseminated organ system involvement. The second stage displays cardiac and nervous system abnormalities as well as arthralgia. Cranial neuropathies, meningitis, radiculopathy, myopericarditis, atrioventricular block, and left ventricular disfunction may be manifested during the second stage of Lyme Borreliosis. The third stage displays chronic mono-or polyarticular arthritis, and/or encephalitis. Rarely, the patient may display chronic atrophic, "tissue paper"-like skin changes of extremities known as acrodermatitis chronica atrophicans.

DIAGNOSIS AND TREATMENT

Because the vast majority of patients have no recollection of a tick bite, patient history of such an event is not helpful. A history of visit to or residence in an endemic area in a patient with appropriate clinical findings is diagnostic in early cases.

Serologic studies for IgM and IgG antibodies against Borrelia Burgdorferi become significantly sensitive in the later part of the first stage of Lyme Borreliosis. A serologic titer done on a patient who displays only primary EM is to poorly sensitive to have any clinical value.

Cultures for B. burgdorferi do exist, but are not available in all areas of the U.S. The culture should be performed on EM lesions. Culture of primary EM is poorly sensitive while that of secondary EM can be nearly 100% in an excellent laboratory.

Skin biopsy of EM is not diagnostic. It is most useful if clinical findings are not convincing and there is a need to rule out other diseases. The CDC definition of Lyme Borreliosis is:

a) Physician-diagnosed EM in a patient who has acquired a definite infection in a geographic area proven to have endemic Lyme Borreliosis.

Or

b) Laboratory evidence of infection with Borrelia and clinical presence of EM in a patient who acquired infection in a geographic area without endemic L.B.

Treatment is dependent on the stage of the disease. Stage I Lyme Borreliosis should be treated with Doxycycline 100 mg orally twice a day or Amoxicillin 500 mg orally three times daily. Patients should remain on the antibiotic for 3 weeks. Amoxicillin at 40 mg/kg/day divided into 3 doses is the choice of drug in children and pregnant women.

If the patient demonstrates stage II of Lyme Borreliosis at presentation without evidence of neurological disease or carditis the above antibiotics may still be employed, but the treatment regimen should be extended to 4–6 weeks in duration. Any patient diagnosed with second or third stage disease who demonstrated neurological or cardiac complications requires a minimum of collaboration with the appropriate specialist. Some of these patients will benefit by referral but are best served by collaboration on a case-per-case basis. These patients usually require treatment with IV antibiotics laftrizone or cefotaxime most commonly and close observation.

MANAGEMENT

To Manage

▾ Keep all first stage and those second stage without neurological or cardiac involvement.

▾ Treatment

lst stage—Tetracycline 100 mg orally BID x 3 weeks *or*

Amoxicillin 500 mg orally TID x 3 weeks

(Children 40 mg/kg/d divided TID)

2nd stage—Same antibiotics as above but treat for 4–6 weeks.

Collaborate at a minimum on 2nd stage disease with neurologic or cardiac involvement, 3rd stage disease, or if patient is pregnant.

▾ Patient education

Remove any tick with forceps placed close to the skin.

Send

Any cases where diagnosis is in question after full work-up in primary care setting.

Cases that do not respond to antibiotic therapy.

Late Stage II and III cases to appropriate specialist which were decided best watched closely during collaboration.

PROGNOSIS

Once antibiotic therapy is initiated, Lyme Borreliosis will begin to resolve within a week. Recurrence is uncommon and treated the same as the initial episode. Concern arises with delay of diagnosis until after neurological or cardiac symptoms develop. These patients may be afflicted with permanent organ-system damage as a result.

PEARLS AND PITFALLS

▾ Collaborate with a specialist if any questions arise.

▾ Pregnant women are treated with Amoxicillin three times daily. Collaborate with the obstetrics service on these patients.

▼ If atrophic skin changes occur in late disease, permanent disfigurement results.

▼ Failure to respond to treatment requires rethinking the entire diagnosis with all useful collaboration. Consider PCR.

▶ ROCKY MOUNTAIN SPOTTED FEVER

BACKGROUND

Rocky Mountain Spotted Fever is the most common and severe rickettsial infection seen in the USA. This potentially fatal illness is spread via the dog tick in the eastern U.S. and the wood tick in the western U.S. The responsible organism, rickettsia rickettsii, is transmitted via these vector Dermacentor ticks within 10 hours of attachment. The regions of the U.S., that are reliably endemic for RMSF include North/South Carolina, Georgia, Virginia, Kansas, Missouri, Montana, Oklahoma, Texas, and New York City. The vast majority of cases occur between April 1st and October 1st, and mostly early in the summer.

In the Clinic

RMSF is associated with a 3–14 day incubation period and a prodrome of malaise, anorexia, and chills occurs. After the prodrome a set of severe symptoms may develop abruptly. These include fever, headache, cough, generalized myalgia, photophobia, nausea, and conjunctival erythema. At approximately day 4 of the illness a characteristic rash appears in the majority of patients. Lesions are erythematous macules and papules which a re blanchable initially but evolve within 5 days to hemorrhagic, nonblanchable and painful. These small ($< \frac{1}{2}$ cm diameter) cutaneous lesions start on the wrists and ankles, appear on the palms and soles and by day 7 centripetally to the trunk and face. Only about 10% of patients never experience a rash. At day 5 to 7 of the illness, multi organ system involvement, becomes apparent. Patients experience high grade fever, abdominal pain, diarrhea, hepatomegaly, splenomegaly, confusion, incontinence, oliguria hypotension, myocarditis, and pulmonary edema.

DIAGNOSIS AND TREATMENT

Rocky Mountain Spotted Fever must be treated very early on your presumptive diagnosis, before all the test results can be analyzed.

This diagnosis may not be clear for weeks, well after the patient has recovered entirely.

CLINICAL FINDINGS

Notice an unusually sudden onset of the triad: fever, severe headache, and rash. In our experience, about half the patients have a cough and abdominal discomfort early in the disease. The rash is at first a toxic erythema on the upper torso, and then changes into crops of painful purpura in bands around wrist and ankles. Larger, very painful lesions soon appear on finger tips. These lesions are emboli of rickettsia from the lung. All of these clinical findings are quickly progressive; the patient is very ill.

Initial laboratory evaluation should include a complete blood count and a chemistry panel. Anemia, thrombotopenia, and slight leukopenia are commonly seen. An elevated BUN and reduced serum sodium are common and indicates renal involvement. The gastrointestinal tract when affected, may manifest via laboratory work-up as an increased alkane phosphate, SGOT, or bilirubin level. Some patient's disease progresses and disseminated intravascular coagulation may develop. Immunofluorescent antibody tests to RMSF specific IgG and IgM are widely employed but requires approximately 10 days for diagnostic titers to be established. Biopsy of skin lesions demonstrate a necrotizing vasculitis and is nonspecific but may help narrow the diagnosis. Immunofluorescence of the biopsied sample may demonstrate R rickettsial antigen. Although immunofluorescence of a biopsied lesion is most helpful tests that can be performed to quickly establish a diagnosis, unfortunately may false negatives will occur. The rickettsii antigen is not universally recognized via this method in all affected patients. Consider PCR.

If left untreated, the fatality rate of RMSF approaches 20%. Death can occur as early as 5 days after the causative arthropod bite usually from pulmonary disease. Treatment reduces the mortality rate to less than 5%. Thus early recognition and prompt initiation of appropriate therapy is key in reducing the morbidity and mortality associated with RMSF.

Treatment of early infection is with oral administration of tetracycline 500 mg four times a day for 7 days of therapy. If the patient is a child over the age of 8, the dose of tetracycline is 50mg/kg/day divided into four doses. In children less than 8 years old or if tetracycline is otherwise contraindicated then intravenous chloramphenicol may be used. The dose is 50 to 75 mg/kg/day given in 4 divided doses with each dose not to exceed 3 grams. If systemic symptoms are significant the patient needs inpatient therapy with intravenous tetracycline at doses of 500 mg four times a day. An alternative intravenous therapy is chloramphenicol at doses of 100 mg/kg divided into four daily doses. Again, antibiotic therapy must be continued for 5 to 7 days. Those severely ill patients will require case-specific treatment of any associated organ system abnormalities.

Physicians and patients residing in RMSF endemic areas must be educated in proper tick removal to minimize transmission of the infection. Also, the clinical presentation and serious possible consequences of their disease needs to be known by any individual residing in, traveling to, or practicing medicine in an endemic region.

MANAGEMENT

To Manage

▼ Keep those clinically evident cases without severe symptoms of systemic illness.

▼ Tetracycline 500 mg orally QID for 5–7 days.

(Children > 8 yrs old—50 mg/kg/d divided QID)

▼ If tetracycline contraindicated (pregnancy/child < 8 y.o)

▼ Chloramphenicol 50–75 mg/kg/d in four divided doses. Max. Dose 3 grams.

▼ Collaborate on all cases kept in primary care setting.

▼ Patient education in endemic areas:

▼ Proper tick removal

▼ Daily skin checks in high risk months

▼ Signs/symptoms of RMSF

Send

▼ Any case where diagnosis is questioned

▼ Any case with systemic symptoms Consider ICU care early.

PROGNOSIS

A noted earlier, if left untreated RMSF has an overall mortality rate of 15–20%. This number decreases to around 5% (less than 1%, in previously healthy patients) if patients are aggressively treated. The prognosis is directly related to the time lapsed before appropriate therapy is initiated and whether or not the patient has recollection of the offending tick bite. The most common complications are seizures, encephalopathy, congestive heart failure, and renal in sufficing.

PEARLS AND PITFALLS

▼ Less than 5% of RMSF patients present with the entire classic triad of fever, rash, and clear history of recent tick bite. Still, 90% are acutely ill with the rash. Early diagnosis depends on the skin signs.

▼ 10% of RMSF patients never display the characteristic cutaneous changes.

▼ Adults (> 16 yrs) experience more severe disease and increased systemic symptomatology than do children. They also are less likely than children to have the rash.

▼ Do not hesitate to immediately collaborate on any case of suspected RMSF.

▼ Remember RMSF *can* occur during fall & winter months and can be seen in non-indigenous regions.

CASE 7.8

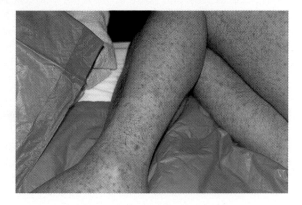

S: A 25-year-old white male presents to your clinic in Fulton, Missouri with complaints of being "sick." When questioned further he sates that he has had a 5 day history of fever up to 103 degrees Fahrenheit, headache, and achy muscles "all over" his body. One day after the above symptoms started he began to experience photophobia and became extremely nauseated. He denies having vomited. He thought it was all part of the "flu or something" and wouldn't have come to the clinic ordinarily. What really brought him to your office today was the onset of a rash 2 days prior to his visit. He states the rash began as small pinkish spots on his wrists and ankles. It then moved to his palms and soles. Finally this morning he noticed it had spread over almost his entire body and had become bright-red in color. You have known the patient his entire life. In fact, you delivered him at the local hospital. You know him to otherwise by very healthy and on no medications. Further questioning reveals a trip to Montana he took a little over a week ago. He was involved in the Glacier Park Mountain Biking Finals in which he took second place. He denies any knowledge of having been bitten by a tick and states he found no such arthropod in any of his clothing. He did spend the 4 days he was in Colorado camping with his girlfriend in a heavy wooded campsite. He denies any other recent outdoor work or recreation. In fact up until he began to feel ill he was working 12 hour days at his job as a physical therapist at the orthopedic clinic in nearby Columbia, Missouri. Further questioning reveals no further pertinent information.

O: A well-nourished, athletic white male who is lacking his usually affable charm. He appears pale and weak. His vital signs show a blood pressure of 115/82 and pulse of 75 while lying flat. When standing his blood pressure is 90/70 and his pulse increases to a rate of 88. His temperature is 103.4 degrees Fahrenheit by mouth. His skin is diaphoretic. It also demonstrates widespread deep red macules without any sign of secondary change. The rest of his physical examination is unremarkable.

A: Rocky-Mountain Spotted Fever

P: Admit the patient to the inpatient service. Begin appropriate IV fluids and antipyretics. Start oral tetracycline at doses of 500 mg four times daily. Watch the patient closely. He may be discharged once he is well hydrated and followed closely as an outpatient. The dose of Tetracycline must be continued for two weeks.

PATIENT EDUCATION HANDOUT
TICK-BORNE DISEASE

Your doctor has diagnosed you with the following disease:_____.

This disease was passed to your body by a tick bite.

It is important to make note of a tick bite when it occurs—keeping the tick may be helpful.

If you find a tick on your skin remove as follows:

—Clean skin around tick with rubbing alcohol. Once dry, use clean forceps (tweezers) and grasp the tick as close to the skin as possible. Pull straight up gently until the tick comes off the skin.

If the tick separates into pieces, proceed to a medical facility for aid in removal.

You may experience some mild swelling, redness, and itching where bitten. These are natural allergic reactions that some people have to tick bites.

If the redness increases around the bite or you feel ill in any manner up to 1 month after a tick bite phone your physician to report the symptoms. They will inform you if you need to be seen.

If you get a red-dot or pimple like a rash on your wrists, ankles, or anywhere else after a tick bite, see your doctor immediately.

Your doctor has prescribed a medicine called_____.
Take all of this medication until it is gone. If you have any problems with the medicine, tell your doctor. Don't even stop without letting the doctor know.

CHAPTER 8

DERMATOLOGY IN SELECT GROUPS

DIABETIC PATIENTS

As primary care physicians we care for many diabetic patients in our practices. Diabetes has a number of associated cutaneous diseases that may develop secondary to the underlying endocrine abnormality. These skin rashes (Table 8.1) are not seen in all patients with a diagnosis of diabetes, but can develop and should be considered if a suspicious lesion arises.

In addition, wounds or skin breakdown in the lower extremities of the diabetic patient may lead to secondary pyoderma and/or a poorly healing wound. The presence of possible associated peripheral neuropathy or small vessel peripheral vascular disease in this subset of the patient population is the accepted pathophysiological mechanism behind these poorly healing lesions. Amputation of digits, feet, or even entire lower limbs may result from a pyoderma in the diabetic patient.

The most common pathognomic cutaneous change associated with diabetes is a form of chronic dermatosis known as *necrobiosis lipiodicum diabeticum*. Although, a diagnosis of diabetes is not essential in the patient with NLD about 70% of individuals with this cutaneous change have a diagnosis of diabetes mellitus. In those patients with diabetes, less than 1% display these lesions. The exact pathophysiology behind presence of NLD is not known. Researchers believe that the lesions arise as a result of microangiopathic changes in blood vessels.

The lesions themselves appear as discrete, well circumscribed yellowish plaques. These plaques are round to oval shaped and often

TABLE 8.1 ▼ Cutaneous Changes and Diabetes Mellitus

Diabetic Bullae
Necrobiosis Lipiodicum Diabeticorum
Diabetic Dermatopathy
Staphylococcal Bacteria Infection
Candidal Yeast Infection
Dermatophyte Infection

have a raised violaceous hued margin. 90% of NLD are found on the anterior tibial areas of the lower legs. Infrequently such lesions can be found on the extensor surface of the arm, the dorsal surface of the feet, or the face. Approximate one-half of patients display the lesions bilaterally.

Palpation of NLD reveals a waxy texture and marked atrophy. The atrophic lesions may breakdown and form subsequent shallow ulcers. These ulcerations should be watched carefully for the possible development of a secondary pyoderma. The vast majority of NLD are asymptomatic but some do have associated burning or pruritus.

The differential diagnosis of NLD includes chronic eczema, pretibial myxedema, and morphea. Usually clinical suspicion is adequate in differentiating these various skin diseases, but if necessary a biopsy is diagnostic. Complications most often arise as a result of secondary bacterial infection and resultant poor healing. Diabetic patients with NLD must be watched closely for such pyodermas and educated in self-examination of these lesions.

Treatment of NLD includes topical mid potency steroid application twice daily with addition of an occlusive dressing to improve efficacy. If one month of topical therapy demonstrates no improvement, intralesional Kenalog may be employed. The injection of steroid does increase the risk of possible ulceration so follow the patient closely. Some physicians use 75 mg to 225 mg of Dipyramidale a day with 325 mg of aspirin every other day in treating the patient with NLD. It is thought that the prevention of platelet aggregation and subsequent small vein thrombosis may improve these cutaneous lesions, but its efficacy has not been shown to date. The majority of NLD can be handled in the primary care setting. Send patient who are not responding to therapy for confirmation of diagnosis. If ulceration occurs and pyoderma develops monitor the patient very closely.

Other less common cutaneous changes may be found in the diabetic patient. These include *diabetic dermatopathy, diabetic bullae,* and *infection.*

Diabetic dermatopathy consists of small, hypopigmented macules with clear margins and little other secondary change. These macules are found almost universally on the lower legs where they arise secondary to trauma. These lesions, like NLD, arise as a result of small vessel thrombosis. No treatment exists, but these macules rarely become complicated and their course is rather benign.

Diabetic bullae are often seen on the ankles and feet of a diabetic patient. These bullae are filled with a clear-yellow serosanguinous fluid. Breakdown of the overlying roof will lead to the formation of an erosion which must be watched closely for pyoderma formation. The exact etiology of these pemphigoid-like lesions is not known, but they appear to arise from normal looking skin. The presence of trauma, ischemic, or infection is not necessary for their formation. Treatment consists solely of close observation for possible secondary infection until the bullae spontaneously resolves. No specific therapy is otherwise indicated.

The propensity for staphylococcus bacterial infections and candidal yeast infections of the skin of the diabetic patient is well known. The patient must be made aware of the importance of reporting any signs or symptoms of such infections immediately so that quick and proper treatment can be employed. Proper patient education is vital in the management of the diabetic skin. We have previously discussed the treatment of bacterial pyoderma in Chapter 6 of this text. Also noteworthy is the effectiveness of oral griseofulvin at doses of 500 mg each day in treating fungal infections of the diabetic. Especially if any associated fissuring or cracking of the skin is present. At a minimum, topical antifungals and Betadine soaks once a day with every other day debridement are necessary adjuncts in these diabetic with a fungal infection.

▶ Diabetic Foot Care

Diabetic foot care is essential in helping prevent lesions that could develop into major health problems due to bad healing in these patients. The following is a guide for the patient that should be emphasized when communicating with a diabetic patient.

1. If you smoke—STOP.
2. Every day closely inspect your feet for cuts, blisters, or other lesions.
3. Have your feet measured each time new shoes are purchased.
4. Every day, before putting shoes on—check the insides for possible foreign objects.
5. Have your physician check your feet at each visit.
6. Never walk bare footed.
7. Keep feet clean and dry.
8. If a callus or corn needs removed—see your podiatrist as physician. DO NOT REMOVE YOURSELF.
9. Buy shoes that lace up and have a wide-toe-box.
10. Do not soak feet in hot water or apply heating pad.
11. Use emollients to keep skin soft daily—this helps prevent cracking and fissuring.
12. Always cut nails straight across—do not "round off" corners.
13. Call your physician immediately if problems, questions, or concerns.

THE NEONATE

There exist several interesting, normal skin changes in the newborn infant. There also occur a handful of dermatological abnormalities which are more serious and deserve mention in this text. But, for the most part the skin findings seen in infants near birth are benign in nature and pose no threat to the overall well-being of the child. Unfortunately, most parents of these children have little experience in diagnosing rashes and are likely to bring their infant into the clinic with any skin change they feel is abnormal.

Sebaceous hypertrophy is very common in the newborn infant. Such gland hypertrophy is mostly seen on the child's face and often on the upper trunk, although it can be found anywhere on the patient's skin. This sebaceous gland hypertrophy can lead to excessive sebum production and a possibly oily appearance to the skin. As a general rule, the sebum production of the average infant is minimal. The baby's skin is frequently insulted by contact with breast milk, formula, urine, and feces. Thus, the environment becomes moisture laden with an increase in sweat retention. In addition, frequent use of thick, ointment emollients to moisturize the infant's skin will lead to occlusion of sweat ducts and follicles and secondary irritation of these structures. This occlusion often causes the formation of *mil-*

iaria. Miliaria are small, white, pustule-like lesions that often cluster in an affected area. Associated inflammation is minimal and rarely is any significant redness associated with these acne-like lesions. Miliaria are commonly referred to as prickly heat. Treatment of these wholly benign lesions consists of parental reassurance, avoidance of thick ointments, and minimizing the moisture-laden environment of the affected skin. Lipid-free cleansers and creams should be employed in routine skin care of the infant. These skin care products will minimize the occlusion of sweat glands and follicles.

Pigmentary abnormalities are common in the newborn as well. About 1 in 200 babies have *cafe-au-lait* marks. These flat, light-brown patches of skin change can range in size from 1 to 10 cm in diameter. They can be solitary or numerous and their distribution on the skin in wholly random. Although commonly present at birth they may appear on the patient's skin through childhood age. These patches of color change become clinically relevant when present in numbers of four or greater. Numerous cafe-au-lait spots are indicative of a tendency to develop neurofibromatosis. Otherwise the lesions themselves are wholly benign and do no show any tendency towards the formation of melanoma. The patient's parents should be educated about neurofibromatosis when indicated but otherwise should be wholly reassured that these lesions require no specific treatment. Infants are not born with *melanocytic nevi*. These macules will begin to develop in early childhood and will continue to appear in crops through the mid-twenties.

Another pigmentary finding in the newborn is exclusive to the black-skinned patient. Some Afro-American babies may be exceptionally *hypopigmented* at birth. In fact, an infant of two black-skinned parents may appear nearly white when born. Their skin color may be strikingly different from their biological parent's skin tone. This normal hypopigmentation is merely a delay in the neonate's development. The baby will darken their skin pigment soon after birth, usually within only a few days. The examiner can look at the skin around the neonate's fingernails where a zone of increasing melanin pigment is found. This area of the baby's skin will display the darkening pigment changes before other areas.

Strawberry hemangiomas are a type of vascular tumor that can be present at birth or develop within the first year of life. These tumors occur in approximately seven percent of infants and are usually singular but may be multiple in number. The vascular lesion begins as a purple-red nodule or telangectasia. Over a few months they rapidly enlarge to form large, easily compressible nodules. These tumors may be as small in diameter as 2 centimeters or as large as 10 centimeters. Their name denotes the typical bright red color of these well demarcated lesions. Strawberry hemangiomas are composed of immature blood vessels clustered together in the dermis. If the immature vessels extend deeper into the subcutaneous tissue the lesion is termed a *cavernous hemangioma*. These deeper vascular tumors appear as single or multiple, ill-defined, purplish-red masses. Cavernous hemangiomas and strawberry hemangiomas have similar prognoses and treatment protocols. As previously mentioned these lesions represent an area of immature cutaneous vascularity. In over 95% of cases, as the patient ages the involved vessels mature. Usually the lesion spontaneously resolves within 5–10 years. Any hemangioma that compresses local vital structures or does not fully remit be age 10 should be referred to a dermatologist or plastic surgeon for appropriate treatment.

Unlike the aforementioned hemangiomas, *port wine stains* will not spontaneously resolve. Unfortunately, these large purple-red patches of skin discoloration represent mature vascular nevi.

Also known as nevus flammeus, these tumors are usually unilateral and can appear anywhere on the infants body. They are always present at birth and do not develop later in life. The appear as well-demarcated, irregularly-shaped, flat patches of skin change. As the patient ages the surface of the port-wine-stain may take on a "cobblestone-like" appearance. These vascular lesions may represent the presence of a neurocutaneous syndrome—either Klippel-Trenaunay-Weber or Sturge-Weber. Port-wine stains present a significant cosmetic problem to the patient as they mature. Often an infant's parents are quite emotionally distressed over the presence of this permanent, disfiguring lesion. Often the color change can be improved with the practiced use of waterproof make-up. Permanent treatment options are limited to removal via laser methods. Although argon and carbon-dioxide laser treatment is quite effective, these methods of removal can leave some resultant scar, are very expensive, and not widely available.

Mongolian spots are areas of dermal melanocytosis. These lesions are seen in 80 to 90 percent of all infants of African-American heritage. Whereas, they manifest themselves in less than 10 percent of Caucasian neonates. Mongolian spots are wholly benign and do not represent any threat to the infant. The spots of hyper melanosis may be seen in infants who also display hemangiomas and/or melanocytic nevi. They are permanent and should never be treated. Attempts at removal are likely to result in scaring that is more cosmetically unfavorable than the original lesion.

Eczema can present a problem to many neonates. Infants commonly manifest only two forms of eczema—atopic dermatitis and irritant contact dermatitis. Both of these forms of eczema were fully discussed in Chapter 6 of this text and will only be briefly mentioned here.

Atopic dermatitis is often the first systemic symptom in an atopic child. Remember that the eczematous skin changes of an atopic individual are merely one portion of the disease process as a whole. In order to be diagnosed as true "atops," patients must have a personal or family history of environmental allergies, asthma, or dermatitis. About 15-20% of the US population has inherited an atopic diathesis, and about 5% have clinical evidence of atopic dermatitis at some point during their lifetimes. Neonates do not show any sign of this skin disease. It does not manifest itself until four to five months of age, even in the most severe cases. About 90% of all patients who develop atopic dermatitis will show the typical skin findings of the disease before the age of 5 years. Onset of atopic dermatitis while in adult life is very rare. The exact pathogenesis of atopic dermatitis is not known. But, researches have demonstrated that IgE serves an important role in the development of this disease process. In fact, a patient with an eczema suspected to be of atopic nature should have a serum IgE level checked. Elevation of serum IgE strengthens the diagnosis of atopic eczema in the patient with generalized eczematous skin changes.

In children atopic dermatitis appears as poorly-marginated, erythematous, micro-vesicular plaques. These skin changes can occur anywhere on the patient, but are most commonly seen over the face, neck, legs (especially the extensor surface of the knees) and in the antecubital fossa of the upper extremities. The disorder is universally intensely pruritic. The pruritus can be severely debilitating and lead to emotional irritability and disturbed sleep, as well as the expected mechanical scratching of the skin. The severe scratching will lead to skin excoriation which f further damages the affected skin. This additional damage induced by scratching in turn, leads to more pruritus. Thus, begins the "itch-scratch cycle" of skin damage associated with this eczematous disease. Management of atopic dermatitis in children is similar to that in the adult patient. Please refer to

Chapter 6 of this text for the details of proper management of atopic dermatitis.

Irritant contact dermatitis is the most common eczema seen in the neonatal patient population. In infants this contact dermatitis is almost universally presents as diaper rash. *Diaper rash* is a macerated form of irritant contact dermatitis and was also thoroughly discussed in Chapter 6 of this textbook. Uncomplicated diaper dermatitis can be controlled reliably simply by improving the moisture-laden environment almost universally present in patients suffering from the skin disease. Unhappily, in severe cases this means not only protective emollients and frequent diaper changes, but actual near total avoidance of diaper use. Gentle cleansing and thorough air drying are vital to the improvement of the skin rash. Infrequently, diaper dermatitis is complicated with a fungal infection. The responsible pathogen is usually candida and the rash takes on the edematous, vesicular, bright red appearance of a typical candidal skin infection.

Seborrheic dermatitis is also common in neonates. This eczema-like skin disease (discussed in Chapter 6) usually affects infants from 2-16 weeks of age. The disease occurs in this age group as an epidermal response to newly activated sebaceous glands. The exact pathophysiology behind its development is not known. Seborrhea in the infant presents as poorly marginated patches of erythematous papules. The areas of skin commonly affected include the eyebrows, hairline, scalp, ears and diaper area. Seborrheic dermatitis of the scalp is colloquially referred to as "cradle cap." Secondary changes of the rash include thick, greasy whitish-yellow scale. The process is not very pruritic and rarely causes the patient any discomfort. Seborrhea in the infant can be quite cosmetically unsightly in its appearance. It is a common dermatological complaint of the parent when presenting to the clinic for early well-child examinations. It can be so unsightly as to be the chief cause of presentation.

Finally, a brief note on the *alopecia* experienced by almost all infants. Newborn babies lose the vast majority of the hair that was present at birth. This alopecia occurs from one to three months after their birth. Although extremely common, the alopecia often goes unnoticed by the parents and care givers. The event may not be noted due to the quick loss of birth hair at the same time new hair in growing in. Interestingly, the alopecia is unnoticed despite a frequent corresponding change in the infant's hair color. If the parent does raise concern over the hair loss they should be thoroughly reassured by the practitioner.

THE PREGNANT PATIENT

Women often experience a variety of skin and hair changes during the course of pregnancy and the post-partum period (Table 8.2). The vast majority of these cutaneous changes are normal and benign although some are cosmetically unsightly. Below a few of these skin changes are outlined.

Pigmentary Changes

Hyperpigmentation can occur suddenly in the pregnant woman. Often this change is manifested as a patchy brown hyperpigmentation of the face, most notably the cheeks. This "mask of pregnancy" is termed melasma or chloasma. It occurs as a result of the deposition of melanin in the sun damaged and hair bearing areas of the face. Local hyperpigmentation of the nipples, axilla, areola, vulva, and the midline of the abdomen (linea alba) can occur and resolve over many months after delivery of the fetus. In addition, nevi may darken a shade or two. Often this darkening is mistaken for a new, or growing, nevus. The concerning mole(s) should be examined closely but the incidence of melanoma is not substantially increased in the pregnant population.

Vascular Changes

Along with pregnancy, various vascular changes occur. The "healthy glow" of pregnancy is one such result of vascular change. In addition, spider telangectasia, varicosities, palmar erythema, and

TABLE 8.2 ▼ Skin Changes in Pregnancy

Hyperpigmentation
Vascular changes
     Spider hemangiomas
     Palmar erythema
     Varicosities
     Hemorrhoids
     Pyogenic granulomas
Nevi (darkening of)
Striae Distensae
Pruritic Urticarial Papules and Plaques of Pregnancy (PUPPP)
Herpes Gestations
Hair Growth

hemorrhoids can occur. Although telangiectasia and varicosities may persist after delivery, most spontaneously resolve with time. Pyogenic granulomas are a benign granulation tissue-like growth that may flourish during pregnancy. These friable tumors may occur in very large numbers. Usually they are seen in the scalp and in various skin fissures. They often occur on the face, and when present, can have an unsightly appearance. These pyogenic granulomas resolve over time with delivery. Often a significant amount of reassurance on the part of the physician is necessary.

Stria distensae are commonly known as stretch marks. These skin changes occur as a result of stretch and hormone induced separations of the reticular dermis. These cutaneous unregularitis are seen most commonly on the thighs and the trunk. Weight gain has been proven to have no effect on the presence or absence of striae. Some women with a 50 pound weight gain won't suffer from these changes while a women who gains a mere 10 pounds will. The vast majority of women find these marks unsightly, most especially when they are present on the breasts. Although many creams and ointments tout the ability to improve stria, no therapy has been proven even minimally effective in reducing their appearance. Almost all stria gradually improve after delivery, at a minimum most fade.

Hair Changes

Often with pregnancy body hair will darken in color. A "mustache" may appear or arm, leg hair will become darker and coarser in nature. Unfortunately, some of this new pigmented body hair will sometimes persist after delivery. This phenomena is most common with linea alba hair and nipple hair but can occur with facial hair as well.

Also, as a general rule, scalp hair will thicken and grow significantly faster during pregnancy. The increased thickness occurs as a result of the suppression of normal telogen cycles. After delivery, the telogen phase returns and hair loss often ensues. In addition, nails will grow at a faster rate as well.

In addition to the numerous normal skin and hair changes experienced during pregnancy, a few abnormal dermatoses can occur. The two most notable forms of abnormal skin change are pruritic urticarial papules and plagues of pregnancy (PUPPP) and herpes gestations (HG).

PUPPP occurs most commonly late in pregnancy usually during the third trimester. It is seen in 1 in 300 pregnancies and its etiology is not known. Also known as toxic erythema of pregnancy, it is more likely to occur in primigravidas with only 25% of cases in multi gravidas. The rash consists of papules and plaques of an urticarial nature which arise initially within abdominal striae. With time, the erythematous lesions will spread to globally involve the abdomen with possible migration to the breasts, chest, back, and the extremities. The lesions are never vesicular and the presence of blisters or bullae requires further investigation. Scrape for scabies; consider a biopsy. PUPPP is very pruritic and the patient usually presents with visible skin excoriations and complaints of itching.

PUPPP will resolve spontaneously within same week of delivery. Due to its limited nature and lack of risk to mother or fetus, treatment of the eruption is conservative. The risks to fetus or the benefit to the mother should always be considered before initiating therapy. Effective treatment includes topical application of mid-potency corticosteroid creams, twice daily along with oral antihistamines every 6-8 hours as needed. Collaborate on diagnosis before using oral steroids. Colloidal oatmeal baths are also often helpful. If the pruritus is severe, than oral prednisone at doses of 20 to 40 mg a day is often helpful.

Herpes Gestations

This rare pruritic rash of pregnancy represents an immunologic incompatibility between mother and fetus and despite its nomenclature, is not related to the herpes virus. HG is less common than PUPPP and only one-third of patients are primigravidas. It can occur at any time during the course of the pregnancy, but the most common time is late second to early third trimester. The lesions arise as a result of an immune mediated phenomenon, notably antibody formation directed against the epidermal basement cell membrane.

The rash itself initially consists of numerous erythematous papules and plaques around the umbilicus which develop into vesicles and bullae within days. Soon, the lesions spread and the entire body may be covered with the fluid-filled lesions. About 5 percent of patients have a rash that appears much like PULP—i.e., without any associated vesicles or bullae. The rash is very pruritic and excoriation with blister roof breakdown is commonly seen.

Diagnosis of HG can usually be based on history and clinical findings, but a small number do mimic PUPPP. If there exists any question in regards to the exceed diagnosis a skin biopsy should be performed to rule out HG. Often referral for this biopsy is appropriate due to the patients usual discomfort and overall apprehension.

HG does not spontaneously resolve after delivery. In fact, cases have been known to persist for more than a year. Also, the rash will often recur in later pregnancies. Some early studies linked HG with fetal death and spontaneous abortion, but more recent investigations have shown only an increased number of premature and low-birth weight deliveries.

Treatment of HG is via oral corticosteroids at doses of 1 mg/kg/day with gradual taper once the rash begins to show signs of improvement. Unfortunately, such systemic steroid therapy an suppress the infants adrenal axis. Thus, the benefit of therapy must be weighed against the risk to the fetus. Topical preparations and oral antihistamines are not effective in treating HG.

Intrahepatic Cholestasis of Pregnancy

This disorder of pregnancy deserves brief mention. Patients complain of generalized itching without primary lesions. Often the examiner will see excoriations as a result of extensive scratching. The pruritus can be severe. Symptoms can begin at any time during pregnancy.

The pruritus occurs as a result of an increase in serum bile acids. Laboratory investigation will show an elevation in cholesterol, alkaline phosphatase, bile acids, and transaminase. There exists no treatment that is at all effective. The only consolation is that all symptoms will stop within 48 hours after delivery. The actual risk to the fetus is not fully understood.

THE ELDERLY PATIENT

As our country's geriatric population continues to grow the demand is increasing for greater knowledge of skin diseases that affect this specific patient population is increasing. Although many dermatologic abnormalities can be found in the elderly patient, certain ones are more prevalent. This text will focus on only those most commonly encountered by the primary care practitioner: pressure sores, generalized poor wound healing, seborrheic dermatitis, hair loss, actinic keratosis and seborrheic keratosis. Although these cutaneous changes can be seen in patients who are not elderly, our intent is merely to make the reader more aware of the greater risk this patient population has of developing these skin disorders.

TABLE 8.3 ▼ Risk Factors for Developing Pressure Ulcers

Neurologic disease
CVA disease
Depression
Drugs affecting sensorium
Fractures
Restraints
Edema
Protein—calorie under nutrition
Bowel Incontinence
Bladder Incontinence

Pressure Sores

By definition a pressure sore is any lesion that arises as a result of unrelieved pressure causing damage of the underlying tissue. Although they can occur at any age, 70% of pressure sores are found in those patients 70 years of age or older. Also known as pressure necrosis or more commonly, bedsores, these cutaneous areas of change are a significant morbidity and mortality factor in the geriatric patient. In fact, a patient with a pressure sore has a 2–6 times greater mortality risk than one with intact skin.

These lesions arise as a result of pressure and friction. A few of the factors which increase the risk of developing pressure ulcers include bed or chair-bound ambulatory status, poor ability to reposition oneself, immobility, incontinence, poor nutrition, and altered level of consciousness. Further risk factors are listed in Table 8.3.

Pressure sores most often occur on the skin overlying bony prominence. Approximately 80% of these wounds are found over the

TABLE 8.4 ▼ Pressure Ulcer Classification

Stage I—Non blanchable erythema of intact skin or discoloration, edema, induration, or warmth over bony prominence.
Stage II—Partial thickness skin loss involving epidermis, dermis, or both. Superficial looks like an abrasion, blister or erosion.
Stage III—Full thickness skin loss involving damage to subcutaneous tissue that extends *down to* (*not through*) the fascia. This ulcer looks like a deep crater.
Stage IV—Full thickness skin loss with extensive destruction, tissue necrosis or damage to muscle, bone, or other supporting structures.

pelvic girdle and the heels. A staging of pressure sores (Table 8.4) from 1 to 4 has been developed and is used widely in the diagnosis and treatment of these lesions. Be certain to remove any overlying eschar so that the wound can be properly staged. Any patient diagnosed with a pressure sore requires a thorough medical work-up for risk factors as previously mentioned. The Braden Scale for Predicting Pressure Sore Risk has been recognized by the Agency for Health Care Policy and Research (AHCPR) and in a widely available and useful tool in the management of these lesions. Treatment of pressure sores is dependent on stage. But first, we wish to reemphasize the importance precaution plays in the management of these wounds.

Patient at risk for the development of pressure sores should undergo whole-body skin examination at least once daily. Skin should be cleansed at any time of soiling and otherwise routinely on an individualized basis. Minimum force and friction should be employed when cleansing. The skin should be kept as moist as possible with the application of moisturizers to dry skin and the minimization of exposure to cold or low humidity. When massaging in moisturizers, only light touch should be used over bony prominence. Attempt to avoid or minimize the time skin is exposed to moisture (incontinence, wound drainage, or perspiration).

Skin injury due to friction or pressure should be minimized. This would include turning, repositioning the patient at least every 2 hours if bed ridden and every 1 hour if chair-bound. Use of foam pillows or wedges to pad bony prominence, minimize on trochanter when side-lying, employing pressure-reducing mattresses/seats, and the use of lubricants, protective films, and dressings. In addition, any possibility for improving the ambulatory steeters of the patient should be investigated and employed if present.

Specific therapy of pressure sores will depend on the stage of the ulceration.

Stage I—pressure sores require no specific dressing. The affected skin should be protected from further injury and should be checked at least once daily.

Stage II—pressure ulcers require a dressing to keep the granulation tissue at the ulcer base moist while allowing the non-affected skin surrounding the wound to be dry. No one moist dressing has been found to be superior to others for this purpose. Any wound dead space can be loosely packed with absorbent dressing material.

Stage III—pressure ulcers have subcutaneous tissue involvement. These ulcers and Stage II ulcers with overlying eschar require surgical debridement, enzymatic agents, autolysis or mechanical removal of prevalent tissue (wet-to-dry dressings, water jets, whirlpool).

Stage IV—pressure ulcers have a high degree of associate mortality. They require extensive surgical exploration and debridement followed by 24 hours of dry dressings and finally moist dressings as above. Prognosis for healing is poor.

All pressure ulcers should be evaluated for infection. Any prevalent drainage necessitates the addition of an oral anti-staph antibiotics. Watch for secondary osteomyelitis or sepsis development. Also, be certain to provide adequate pain control. And, never forget the psychological issue of depression that often develops in the patient with pressure ulcers.

Although pressure sores are not a difficult diagnosis to make clinically, the management of at risk patients and the subsequent treatment if an ulcer develops is laborious. Prevention is the key to managing these skin diseases.

Generalized Poor Wound Healing

Often your elderly patients will complain of the difficult time they have getting their wounds to heal properly. This problem is especially notable in the legs. The primary etiology for this increase in time-to-wound-healing is the poor mico-circulation that eventually develops as one becomes more aged.

It is really not concerning that a cut or scrape takes longer to heal until we consider the increased time these wounds have to develop secondary pyodermas or fungal infections. Thus, be certain to stress the importance of regular use of topical antibacterial on cuts or scrapes as well as immediate visits to the physician for any deeper, more serious skin wounds. Patients should be educated on the early signs of infection and the importance of early physician intervention. Prevention and close observation are keys in working with the poor wound healing experienced by the elderly patient.

Seborrheic Dermatitis

Chapter 6 of this text addressed seborrheic dermatitis at length. It is rementioned here because this disease becomes more prevalent with increasing age. Many elderly patients with a history of seborrheic will see a worsening of the condition. Others who have never been afflicted will come to develop the disease. Treatment and management of seborrheic is no different in the elderly patient than in any other age group. Remember that the more severe the skin changes the longer the treatment course warranted.

Hair Loss

Alopecia, or hair loss, was previously addressed in Chapter 7. As the patient ages the ratio of the rate of hair growth to hair loss is decreased. Total body thinning of body hair occurs. Thus, pubic and axillary hair becomes more sparse just as scalp hair becomes thinner. Often times though the rate of hair loss may be more severe. Eyebrows, hair in ears and in arms may increase.

These greater rates of hair loss are often associated with the presence of systemic illness, (such as anemia, thyroid disease, cancer) which is more likely to develop as one ages. Also, the elderly patient is more likely to be taking medication on a regular basis and, thus, is at a greater risk of ingesting a drug that can cause alopecia as a side effect. Hair loss due to abnormal scalp skin as a result of psoriasis and seborrheic dermatitis is more common in the older patient. These etiologies of alopecia all cause diffuse hair loss. Alopecia areata is quite rare in the elderly patient population. The treatment of hair loss is dependent on the exact etiology. Thus, the physician must first determine the cause of the alopecia and then direct therapy accordingly.

Actinic Keratosis

Actinic keratosis (AK) is a form of heliosis or skin changes induced as a result of overexposure to the sun or UVB-light sources. Although heliosis occur in all ages, the effects of sun damage to the skin becomes more apparent as a patient ages. One of the manifestation of this sun exposure is actinic keratosis. These lesions commonly known as "pre-cancers" manifest themselves as discreet, skin changes which is more easily palpated than visualized. They can enlarge to form cutaneous horns of scale. They are seen as a "roughness" of the skin.

Actinic keratosis occurs along with other actinic damage includ-ing wrinkling, elastosis, and epidermal atrophy. Actinic keratosis are most commonly found in areas easily exposed to sun. These areas that are most afflicted are the forehead, cheeks, bald scalp, lower lip, ears, dorsum of hands, and forearms. Any patient with a history of exposure to the sun such as Southern climate, outdoor work, or fair skin is more prone to develop AKs. Although very few AKs will ac-tivate change to squamous cell carcinoma (Chapter 8) a definite ten-dency to do so has been demonstrated. Thus, early and proper treat-ment is essential. Cryotherapy for 10–20 seconds is quick and an efficient method of treatment when dealing with acceptable number of lesions. When sun damage is severs and numerous AK's are pres-ent, treatment with topical 5-Fluorouracil is indicated. This topical agent has better results and more time-effective than attempting cryotherapy on numerous lesions. These patients and 5-FU treat-ment are best handled via referral to a dermatologist.

Seborrheic Keratosis

These benign tumors do not appear until approximately age 30 and they become larger in both size and number as a patient ages. The le-sions begin as small papules with little or no color which enlarge cir-cumferentially and darken over time. Eventually they develop into brown to black, 1 to 5 cm plaques with warty surfaces. The lesion ap-pears almost "stuck on" and close examination reveals a "greasy" texture. The individual lesions are discrete and widely scattered over the face, upper extremities, and trunk.

Treatment of seborrheic keratosis is not necessary unless the le-sion is in an area where it undergoes frequent trauma. If the above scenario is the case, or if cosmetic removal is desired, cryotherapy for 15–20 seconds is nearly universally effective. Individual lesions, once properly treated, rarely recur.

In conclusion, the geriatric population suffers from a number of skin diseases seen less commonly in the younger patient. Entire texts have been devoted to geriatric dermatology. This chapter was in-cluded as a mere over view of a few of the more common skin dis-eases in this patient population.

THE ATHLETE

As the interest and participation in sports and recreational exercise continues to increase, so does the incidence of related skin diseases

(Table 8.5). The physician needs to be aware of these skin changes, their relation to a certain activity or piece of equipment, and their best method of prevention or treatment. The most common inciting etiologies of skin diseases in athletes include moisture, prolonged occlusion, repetitive friction or impact, brief (but severe) impact, allergy to equipment, infections spread by contact with other players, and exposure to wind, heat, and cold weather conditions.

These skin changes are managed by the athletic trainers and team physicians at college and professional level sporting activities. But, it is the primary care physician who is often called upon to treat the athlete that participates at the community or personal level. An athlete's performance can be significantly hampered by various skin abnormalities. The athlete who is educated correctly by their physician has a better change of managing their skin care successfully and will play their sport better and with fewer injuries. Thus, educating the patient on prevention and early intervention of skin disease is a necessary effort on the part of the primary care physician. Sports dermatology is one example of how sports medicine must go beyond just orthopaedics in the proper management of the athletes overall health. Make skin care a regular part of sports medicine.

Dermatologic disease in the athletic population is best approached via an initial breakdown into four general categories. These include the climate induced injury, those with mechanical etiologies, infections, and finally steroid-related skin disease (Table 8.4).

The climate related injuries include frostbite and sunburn. *Sunburn* and various other heliosis are frequently encountered in the athletic population. Runners, triathletes, crew members are among the most commonly afflicted. The best treatment is prevention via a good, waterproof sunscreen with an SPF of at least 15. This number reflects the amount of time the individual will take to burn as compared to exposure without protection. Thus, an SPF of 15 means that the athlete can remain in the sun 15 times longer before burning than if they were wearing no sunscreen. If a patient does sustain a burn then treatment with rest, cool water or Burow's solution compresses, antihistamines, and topical moisturizers is indicated.

Frostbite is often encountered in the athlete as well. High altitudes, cold weather sports such as skiing, are when the perils of frostbite are the greatest. The topic of frostbite was covered in Chapter 8 in greater detail; please refer to this portion of the text. As with sunburn, the best management of frostbite is via prevention. The athlete who chooses to expose themselves to cold temperatures and windy conditions especially at high altitudes, must be well versed in the prevention of cold damage to their skin via proper dress, and frequent rewarming.

Mechanical skin injury is frequently encountered in the athletic population and covers a broad range of dermatologic findings including blisters, corns, calluses, talon noir, green hair, allergic contact dermatitis, acne mechanica, and subungual hematomas.

Blisters can be a very annoying and painful skin finding in almost any athlete. Retained moisture, most often sweat, and friction are the most common contributing factors to the formation of these lesions. Moisture all over the affected skin increases stickiness enough to separate the epidermis from the underlying subcutaneous tissue when an appropriate degree of friction is applied. Fluid collects in the space that forms from this disadhesion and a blister arises. These blisters are often extremely painful and can lead to short-term dehabilitation and the mobility of an athlete to perform at their usual level. Any blister should be drained 3 times in the first 24 hours via a small, clean incision, padded appropriately, and left alone to heal. Any activity that aggravates the healing lesion should be discontin-

TABLE 8.5 ▼ Skin Disease and the Athlete

Climate Induced Injury
Sunburn
Frostbite
Mechanical Injury
Blisters
Corns
Calluses
Talon Noir
Green Hair
Piezogenic Papules
Allergic contact Dermatitis
Acne Mechanica
Subungual Hematoma
Infectious
Dermatophytosis
Herpes Gladiatorum
Keratolysis
Plantar Warts
Steroid-Related Skin Disease

ued until the pain resolves. The blister should *never* be intentionally fully unsoared. This action will result in a severely painful lesion with an increased likelihood of developing a secondary pyoderma.

Blisters are best managed via prevention. The athlete should be encouraged to wear two pairs of socks. One pair being of cotton material while the other polypopalene. This double layer of differing materials allows for the wicking of moisture away from the skin. If heavy sweating is expected a change of socks is often advantageous. Also, when a new sport or pair of shoes is first encountered, it is best to slowly break oneself into activity. This approach gives the skin the time necessary to form protective calluses and reduces the incidence of blister formation.

Calluses are merely hypertrophied, keratinized layers of skin that arise over areas of frequent skin trauma. Again, these lesions serve a protective function. Rarely they will be painful. If pain occurs, limit activity. The callus can be cautiously and conservatively pared down. Plantar warts are often present under a painful callus. Thus, the distinctive tiny black dots of the thrombosed capillary loops of a plantar wart should be sought if a callus is painful enough to require a reduction in size. Calluses that cause no pain should be left alone. Their formation serves an important protective function.

Corns also are areas of keratinized skin cells. These lesions are distinctively shaped as hard, conical structures. They also arise over areas of trauma and are almost exclusively seen on the feet. Corns are exquisitely tender and can be quite debilitating. The best treatment is via the reduction of friction. Padding, changing footwear, and reduction in activity, will all aid in resolution. Choosing an athletic shoe with a wide toe box is an effective method of prevention. Surgical removal is extremely painful and requires a long time course before return to full activity.

Plantar warts are actually not mechanical in their etiology. Rather these painful foot lesions arise as the result of a viral skin infection on the plantar surface. These warts are mentioned here due only to the importance of their similarity to corns, calluses, and blisters. Unlike calluses, plantar warts are painful. Corns we typically conical in shape and do not have the broad, callused appearance of plantar warts. Often a callus lies over the plantar wart. As previously mentioned, the callus should be pared down until tiny black dots are seen. These dark spots represent thrombosed capillary loops. Now the wart can be effectively treated with cryotherapy for 20-30 seconds.

After cryotherapy the wart should be kept well padded and rechecked in two weeks. If any callus reforms it must again be pared away. If the wart persists it must be retreated. Recalcitrant plantar warts may be referred to the dermatologist for DNCB therapy.

Any sport that requires repetitive pounding of the feet against a hard surface may produce *talon noir*. Talon noir is the term employed to describe small, dappled or linear black areas of skin color change on the heel of the athlete's foot. The color change arises from tiny hemorrhage between the dermis and epidermis induced by a traumatic repetitive shearing force. Talon noir is never painful and requires no treatment. It's only diagnostic importance lies in distinguishing it from melanoma. Once melanoma is clinically ruled out, the athlete should be reassured and no limitation of activity is necessary.

Another skin change that arises from repetitive trauma during heel strike are *piezogenic papules.* Unlike talon noir, these lesions are exquisitely painful. The repeated trauma leads to hernicetion of fat and fibrous tissue through the dermis along the sides of the heel. These outcroppings of subcutaneous tissues are very painful, and severely limit activity. Unfortunately, piezogenic papules are untreatable. Usually the athlete is permanently disabled and cannot return to full, pre-injury activity level. Patient education of realistic treatment expectations is essential.

A brief mention of *green hair* is necessary. This color change is experienced by those swimming who have white, grey, or blond hair. Although the green tint occurs while swimming in pools, it is not a result of the chlorine content of the water. Rather, the color change is induced by copper. Copper salts can leak from the pipes that feed water into a swimming pool. This mineral is easily absorbed by the hair shaft and imparts an odd grey-green color to lighter shades of hair. Treatment is via use of a swim cap or discontinuance of water sports in pools with a high percentage of copper salt present.

Allergic contact dermatitis (ACP) was thoroughly discussed in the chapter on eczema (Chapter 6). It is important for any physician who deals frequently with an athletic population to be made aware of the common occurrence of various types of ACD in these patients. The rubber found in snorkels, fins, and protective pads is a frequent insulting agent. Various chemicals use to treat leather goods may be irritating. Hunting, fishing, and other outdoor activities may lead to exposure to poison oak or poison ivy. The list of potential allergic agents is extensive. If ACD is suspected, the questionable material must be removed from contact with the patients skin. If the etiology cannot be easily determined than referral for patch testing is often appropriate. Topical steroid creams of mid-potency strength applied twice daily an be useful in spreading up resolution of the rash. Oral antihistamines can relieve any associate pruritus. Rarely, if ever, are oral steroids necessary in treating ACD and should be avoided unless facial or genital regions are involved.

The athletic population, especially those that require tight-fitting, padded uniforms (football, hockey) are prone to developing *acne mechanica*. This follicular skin disorder resembles acne vulgaris, but arises from friction and hidrosis and has no bacterial component to its etiology. The occlusive nature of helmets and pads along with the friction they cause to the underlying skin during activity will lead to small, erythematous papules in a follicular pattern. The forehead, occiput, posterior neck, shoulders, and thighs are regions prone to developing acne mechanica. The lesions usually resolve during the off season when the occlusion is no longer present. Treatment is unlike acne mechanica. Reduction of occlusion via wearing a layer of protective fabric, such as a cotton T-shirt, and prompt removal of equipment is often helpful. Regular showering after practice or play with a mildly abrasive loofah or sponge is useful as well. In the dark-skinned athlete the changes can become severe enough if prolonged and keloids can occur.

Subungual hematomas are also a result of repetitive trauma to the feet. Here the toes sustain frictional forces which lead to a separation of the toenail from the underlying nailbed. The resultant space fills with blood and the nail appears dark brown to black in color. The great toes are most commonly affected. Sports with quick starts and steps are those that usually lead to the formation of subungual hematomas in the athletic patient population. These lesions are rarely painful. But, if acutely tender, they may be drained via electrocautery through the nailbed. Release of the collected blood usually allows for a significant reduction in pain. Interestingly, runners usually develop subungual hematomas on the great toe of their dominant foot while tennis players are more commonly afflicted on the non-dominant side.

Infections are the final group of major skin diseases suffered by the athletic patient population. The most common infections are dermatophytid and viral in origin. These skin diseases will be mentioned briefly below.

Dermatophyte infections flourish in the moisture-laden, occlusive environment of the athlete's skin. The hidrosis and resultant maceration are a perfect set-up for invasion by fungal organisms. Tinea pedis and tinea cruris are not colloquially termed "athletes foot" and "jock itch" for no reason. The details on diagnosis and treatment of dermatophytosis was fully explained in Chapter 6 and the reader should refer to these pages for the specifics. Prevention of dermatophyte infections is the most effective form of management of such skin disease. Keeping skin dry via frequent changing of sweaty clothes and socks is a key component of prevention. Also minimizing the use of borrowed towels, jock straps, and other fomites is essential. Many athletes wear rubber sandals while showering to minimize the transfer of dermatophytes. Thus prevention again is important in managing another athletic skin disease. Educating your patients is always important so they can learn the importance prevention plays in the development of dermatophyte infections of the skin.

Herpes simplex infections are extremely common in wrestlers and have been termed *herpes gladiatorum*. These herpes infections pose a problem to the athlete, for the rules of the sport forbid tournament wrestling if any lesions are present. Skin checks are routinely performed prior to the onset of competition. The herpes simplex rash is typical for the disease with clustered groups of erythematous vesicles on an erythematous base. The affected body regions of wrestlers include those areas exposed to the most trauma during the sport. These regions conclude the face, shoulders and upper back. Interestingly, numerous studies have demonstrated that breakouts on most wrestlers are due to reactivation of an athletes *own* herpes infection via the trauma of the sport. This concept is in conflict with the commonly held belief that wrestlers are transmitting the virus between each other during activity. Treatment of any athlete with a herpes simplex infection is via the oral administration of valacyclovir or famciclovir. These agents are most successful if given within 24 hours of the outbreak of the rash. Dosing was detailed in Chapter 6 of this text. It is common practice to initiate prophylactic herpes simples treatment prior to major tournaments. The wrestlers are given the chosen antiviral agent for 6 days before the event. This practice is highly successful and almost universally employed.

Keratolysis occurs as small pits on the plantar surface of the feet. These pits are usually infected with corynebacterium and arise as a result of a chronic, hot, moisture-laden environment. An athletes sweaty, occlusive foot conditions are favorable for keratolysis. One further diagnostic clue is the extremely foul odor that this disease imparts to the affected athlete's feet. The painless pitting is otherwise not bothersome. Treatment is accomplished via removal of the moisture-rich environment. Frequent sock changes and employing 2 pairs of absorbent socks are commonly and successful treatment methods. Here again, patient education is the key to successful disease management.

Finally, we would like to briefly mention the *skin effects of anabolic steroids*. There has been an exponential increase in the use of these drugs in both men and women in sports. In men, skin manifestations include sudden flares of inflammatory acne. The acne lesions arise in odd locations atypical for acne vulgaris. Common sites are the shoulder, chest, thighs, and past auricular areas. Skin signs of injection sites are known as "pops" and are usually easily seen by the examiner. Women who use anabolic steroids have increased acne as well as growth of facial hair. In addition, feminine fat pads are usually lost. Anabolic steroids are dangerous and significantly physiologically altering drugs. Their effects on the athletes body go way beyond these simple skin manifestations. It is noteworthy that the skin findings of anabolic steroids are the initial changes seen in an athlete that is using these drugs.

BLACK SKIN

Afro-Americans in the United States have 35 readily distinguishable shades of color of black skin. This does not even include those more subtle pale colors seen in mixed race persons. Most black-skinned individuals of the world live in subtropical and tropical regions. In these areas the majority of skin diseases are infectious in origin. In this text the focus will be on those diseases seen in our patient population in the United States. Here the tropical diseases such as tuberculosis, yaws, pinta, or chromomycosis are too rare to discuss.

A myriad of myths have surrounded the incidence of certain skin diseases in whites versus blacks and the poor versus the wealthy. Fortunately, most of these notions have been disproved. For a given economic level and life-style there exist very few differences between the incidence of various dermatological disorders in blacks and whites. The races do differ in regards to follicles and hair, but not in sebaceous output, hidrosis, heat tolerance, or ease of injury. The remaining dermatologic differences are likely hereditary coincidences.

The hair follicle in the black patient differs from that seen in the white patient. One obvious result is the distinct effect on hair type and appearance. The black hair follicle produces a flat, helical, tightly curled hair. In addition to the production of a distinctive hair type, the black hair follicle is larger and imparts more of a follicular pattern to many common skin diseases. These same skin abnormalities lack such a pattern in the white-skinned patient whose hair follicles are smaller and less prominent. For example, discoid lupus erythematosus is a deeper, more scarring follicular disease in blacks than in whites. Similarly, pyodermas, pityriasis rosacea, atopic eczema, and psoriasis may be strikingly follicular in the black population. Look for such a pattern to aid in the diagnosing these skin diseases in blacks—do not allow the follicular nature of such rashes throw off your diagnostic skills.

The common occurrence of keloids and hypertrophic scarring in black patients is due to hereditary coincidence. This belief is supported by the tendency of such scarring only in select families, rather than in the black population as a whole. Thus, keloids and hypertrophic scarring tend to be more common in select families of Afro-Americans, and of other races too, including the most fair skinned.

Keloids are more commonly encountered in females than in the male population and are more frequently formed in the pubertal years. These unsightly growths arise around traumatized skin. They grow across the limit of injury and form claw-like extensions of tumorous, hypertrophic tissue. Certain body regions are more prone to form keloids. These include the earlobes (pierced ears), shoulder, and chest. Keloids persist after formation and do not regress or improve with time. These lesions may be a cosmetic nightmare for patients. Unfortunately, they have been shown to be resistant to all forms of therapy including surgery. Often collaborative management is helpful for patient reassurance.

Unlike keloids, hypertrophic scars are not untreatable. These abnormal keratinized wounds are usually limited to the area of injury and also not invade normal, surrounding skin. They often shrink over time even without any treatment. Surgical excision is the treatment method of choice for hypertrophic scars. Surgery almost always leads to a cure.

Skin diseases which manifest with hypopigmentation are a greater concern for those black skinned patients than the white skinned individual. Albinism is the most severe and cosmetically debilitating of all the hypopigmentary disorders. Vitiligo is as common in those with dark skin as those lighter skinned people, but the disease is much more noticeable in the former population. In fact, vitiligo can be cosmetically disfiguring in blacks. Unfortunately, this hypopigmentary skin disease has no effective treatment. Thus, the psychological effects of vitiligo can be severe in the dark skinned patient.

The higher cell content of melanin in the black-skinned patient does provide an increased protection from most heliosis. The incidence of sunburn, photo aging, and epidermal skin tumors (including melanoma) is greatly reduced over the white skinned population. Interestingly though, the rate of photo toxic and photo allergic reactions is equal in those with black skin and those with white skin.

A few additional skin diseases that are more commonly encountered in those with black skin deserve brief mention. These include dermatosis papulosa nigra, perifolliculitis capitis, and the skin findings associated with sickle cell anemia.

Dermatosis papulosa nigra (DPN) is the term employed for a specific type of facial seborrheic keratosis. This seborrheic keratosis are very tiny and dark brown to black in color. They are discrete, well demarcated and appear "stuck-on" as do all seborrheic keratosis. DPN usually arise early in adult life. The lesions are almost exclusively found on the patients face, usually clustered in groups around the eyes and in a "butterfly" pattern on the cheeks. DLN are almost never seen in Caucasians or lighter skinned races. Any attempt at removal will leave an area of depigmentation of similar size as the original lesions. These subsequent, multiple areas of depigmentation are no more beneficial cosmetically than the original lesions. DPN are best left alone. Be certain to educate the patient so realistic results are understood.

Perifolliculitis capitis is an acne form disorder seen exclusively in the dark-skimmed patient. This disorder is usually encountered in young, black males. Perifolliculitis is seen on the scalp and upper neck of these young men as a result of a shattering of the hair shaft itself deep within the follicle. Although the skin changes of perifolliculitis appear similar to grade four acne, this disease is infectious. The shattered hair shaft produces a severe foreign body reaction within the follicle and a subsequent staphloccocal infection. Treat for pyoderma as needed. The pyoderma can spread and a dissecting cellulitis of the scalp usually results. Perifolliculitis capitis often leads to alopecia and keloid formation. A milder form of perifolliculitis can be seen in the beard area of the face. In fact, over one-half of black men have some degree of this mild, beard-area variant. Like its capitis cousin, this form of perifolliculitis results from hair-shaft rupture within the follicle and a secondary staphloccocal infection. Perifolliculitis capitis usually requires surgical management and all patient should be referred to a dermatologist for this procedure. Perifolliculitis in the beard area can be treated via discontinuation of shaving and manual removal of imbedded hairs.

Finally, sickle cell anemia often manifests with dermatologic findings and deserves mention in this chapter. These skin lesions are seen in children and adolescents only. Children may present with the hand-foot syndrome. This term refers to small infarctions in the blood vessels of the hands and the feet of the sickle cell patient. These infarctions lead to a painful, non-pitting edema of the skin over the hands and feet. Often the patient experiences associated fever. Adolescents may have a different dermatologic manifestation of their sickle cell disease. The abnormal red blood cells cause total obstruction of the blood vessels in the lower extremities. These blocked vessels eventually give rise to non-healing leg ulcers. These sickle-cell associated dermatologic diseases are best managed via referral to a specialist unless the primary care physician is well versed in the skin management of this patient population.

▶ Nutrition and the Skin

MALNUTRITION

Whenever patients do not eat an adequate diet or properly digest and absorb the food they have ingested they "starve" their skin as well as their body. Malnutrition can arise from elective reduction of adequate caloric intake as well as from a disease process that leads to a patient's physical inability to eat or to make use of the food that they have ingested. Malnutrition denies the body of essential nutrients. The skin, like other organs of the body, is affected by the loss of calories and nutrients.

The primary effect of malnutrition on the skin is seen as an *inability to repair* itself properly after sustaining injury. Cuts, scrapes, and other insults take a long period of time for adequate healing and frequently form scars. The skin in general becomes thinner, less elastic and more fragile. Bruises appear to form with even the mildest of injuries. Importantly, the mouth, lips and other mucous membranes are areas of the skin that, in a well-nourished state require much faster repair. Thus, these areas show the most damage at the earliest time in the disease course. Also in malnutrition the mouth is sore in general and *perleche* can appear. The skin's normal healthy color is lost and in its place a *dull, sallow color* develops. The malnourished patient has abnormalities of the hair and nails as well as the skin. Not only is hair growth severely retarded, but diffuse *alopecia* often occurs as well. The hair shaft enters a telogen phase which causes the affected hair to fall out of its follicle. In addition, *nails* can become weak, pitted, ridged and fragile.

In addition to the above mentioned general changes in the appearance of the skin, hair, and nails, various specific rashes are associated with malnutrition. *Keratosis pilaris* can form on the face neck, and extremities. The malnutritioned state leads to hyperkeratosis of the skin that surrounds the follicles. This rash appears as small, flesh-colored papules in a follicular distribution over the skin. What results is a "toad skin" look. *Pigmentary changes* can lead to the formation of a rash on the face and neck. This hyperpigmentation occurs in a chloasma-like pattern and leads to extreme cosmetic concern on the part of the patient.

OBESITY

Obesity is quickly becoming one of our nation's greatest risk factors for the development of serious disease. In fact, it is considered a disease by today's medical community. Obese individuals have difficulty with thermoregulation and have a tendency to easily overheat. As a result they often have problems with *flushing* of their skin and excessive sweating *(hyperhydrosis)*. The excess moisture that results from the hyperhidrosis acts in concert with the occlusive nature of multiple body folds of fat to causes maceration. The macerated skin is at greater risk of developing irritant contact dermatitis (Chapter 6) including intertrigo. Also the moisture laden epidermis encourages the formation of *bacterial and fungal skin infections.* In general, all *eczema,* if present, is worse in skin folds. Thus, these grossly overweight individuals will have more serious cases of eczematous disease due to their preponderance of fatty skin folds.

Also, obesity is a significant risk factor for the development of adult-onset diabetes mellitus as well as generalized atherosclerosis of arteries. Both of these serious, life-threatening diseases can lead to peripheral vascular disease and/or congestive heart failure. A symptom of both PVD or CHF is the formation of another type of eczema, *stasis dermatitis.* Thus, obesity is a disease which typically demonstrates an increase in the aforementioned skin diseases over the general, non-obese patient population.

Vitamin A and Carotene

A deficiency of vitamin A is brought on only extreme cases of malnutrition. A patient's resistance to developing vitamin A deficiency results from large, natural, body stores of this nutrient. Thus the disease is almost never seen in non-third-world nations. Interestingly, in the United States, overdoses of vitamin A are much more common than deficiencies of this nutrient. Excess serum levels of vitamin A can lead to headache and various skin abnormalities. These skin changes include generalized xerosis (dryness) with fine, white scaling. The xerosis gives rise to a moderate amount of pruritus and excoriations are commonly found. A diffuse alopecia is common as the hairs are sent into a telogen phase of growth.

Infrequently, a practitioner will encounter a patient who has been ingesting too much carotene and develops characteristic pigmentary changes of certain areas of their skin. Carotenemia refers to a yellowish-orange discoloration of the skin. The yellow appearance arises when blood levels of carotene reach about 4 times normal. Also, at these serum levels, carotene is excreted in the sweat. This excreted carotene is then absorbed into the stratum corneum of the skin. Thus, the palms, soles, elbows, knees, chin and nose all appear bright yellow in color. This nutritional abnormality is quite uncommon and is almost exclusively the result of fad dieting on the part of the patient. Other that the obvious cosmetic affects, such overdoses of carotene are harmless. In fact, the pigmentary changes are actually beneficial in preventing heliosis.

Vitamin E

No convincing evidence exists that a deficiency or abundance of ingested vitamin E affects the human skin in any manner.

Water Soluble B Vitamins

In this country, pellagra is rarely encountered anymore. The few cases that occur are in alcoholics and psychotic patients. In order for pellagra to occur, the patient's diet must be poor in protein, tryptophane, and niacin. Pellagra begins with symptoms of watery diarrhea. Later on in the disease course skin changes develop. These cutaneous manifestations include a typical photo dermatitis which gradually worsens into a brown, scaling eczema. The rash is seen especially over the nose and/or the dorsal surface of the hands. General signs and symptoms of malnutrition are always present with skin signs of pellagra.

Deficiency of thiamin, riboflavin, or pyridoxine can initially induce a painful mouth, scaling lips, and oral perlesche. These skin manifestations can be followed by a eruption that mimics seborrheic dermatitis (Chapter 7). This rash is seen around eyes, nose, ears, mouth and genital regions. But the skin changes associated with a deficiency of water-soluble B vitamins are always associated with some degree of mental status change. This nutritional disorder does respond to therapy with vitamin supplementation which should be initiated immediately. Quite often severe alcoholism is the etiology of the malnourished state.

Iron Deficiency and Excess

Iron deficiency is a nutritional disorder that almost always induces skin changes. These abnormal skin findings include generalized poor healing of wounds and a preponderance of eczematous skin disorders. Hair loss, chronically thin hair, and fragile, thin, flat fingernails are other dermatologic manifestations of iron deficiency. Severely low levels of serum iron may be associated with fragile mucous membranes leading to easy bleeding of gums, a smooth tender tongue, and possibly even a persistent angular stomatitis with deep fissuring. General essential pruritus and ichthyosis like dryness of the entire skin is also seen with the more severe forms of iron deficiency. The vast majority of these cases will respond in time with iron replacement therapy.

An excess of serum iron will lead to dermatologic findings in about 1 in 200 people. These individuals have inherited a tendency to deposit excess iron in the skin. This cutaneous deposition of iron is part of the systemic disease known as hemochromatosis. Early in the course of this disease, the skin assumes an unnatural grey-metal look as a result of iron deposition. As time goes by melanin is deposited in the skin as well and a more bronze pigmentation appears. The diagnosis is reached via clinical findings, laboratory investigation, and skin biopsy.

Zinc Deficiency

The skin relies on a variety of zinc-metal enzymes. Acquired deficiency of zinc is commonly seen in alcoholics but is otherwise rarely encountered in western countries. The first cutaneous sign of zinc deficiency is a severe perleche. This perleche worsens into a vesicular eruption over the eyelids, face and behind the ears. At the same time, erosions develop on the affected patient's fingertips, feet, knees and elbows. The perianal and genital skin may be involved as well in adults. Hair loss almost universally occurs and is a diffuse pattern. Corneal dystrophy can occur and, in certain cases, may become quite severe. A thorough examination of the eye is recommended, even in the milder cases.

A similar disease, acrodermatitis enteropathica, occurs in infants. This abnormality results from the inheritance of a poor intestinal capability to absorb zinc. In this nutritional disorder, low serum levels of zinc lead to reduction in the amount of various zinc-sensitive enzymes that are found in normal skin. The lack of these cutaneous enzymes will lead to the characteristic dermatologic abnormalities. Acrodermatitis enteropathica is quite rare and will not be discussed at any further length here for it is quite uncommon.

Scurvy

Scurvy is seldom seen in modern patient populations, expect in alcoholics and demented people. The body requires only 10 mg of ascorbic acid each day to prevent scurvy from occurring. If present, scurvy manifests a typical set of clinical signs and symptoms. The common clinical picture of scurvy includes lethargy, fatigue, generalized arthralgias, easy bruising of the skin with even mild trauma, and tiny purpura along pressure lines such as beneath the belt or bra straps. One test of easy bruising is the Rumple-Leedes procedure. This test involves the use of a common blood pressure cuff. The cuff is places around the patient's upper arm, inflated, and left in place for 2 to 3 minutes. If the patient has a tendency towards easy ecchymosis formation, removal of the cuff will demonstrate many small petechia over the skin that was compressed.

Severe cases of scurvy involve even further clinical changes. These include mental status changes, visual deficiencies, bleeding gums, pallor, anemia, spreading scars, alopecia, cork-screw hairs with purpura at the base and poor immune response to combating common infections. Alcoholics may develop scurvy rapidly with profound mental changes and florid skin signs.

CHAPTER 9

SPECIAL TESTS AND STUDIES

WOOD'S LIGHT

One usefulness of this light is to see patches of melanin on the skin, which would be scarcely visible in room light. Actinic poikiloderma shows up, as do Café-au-lait spots in neurofibromatosis. This function has been done with only a low-intensity lamp. The second use is to fluoresce diagnostic substances, and for this use, you need a much stronger lamp. You can see some porphyrins (orange-red), products of two bacteria—Cornybacterium minutissima (orange spots of erythrasma) and pseudomonas (yellow-green spots) as well as topical drugs (tetracycline).

Wood's light is not useful to locate or diagnose tinea of the scalp. The organism that now causes 99% of these cases (T. tonsierans) is not fluorescent.

Use the Wood's light in a dark room after you have dark adapted your vision. Hold the light close to the target, but pointed away from your line of vision. Experience is needed because many substances fluoresce, including fabrics, dyes, bath soaps, and medications. Semi-quantitative judgements are possible as in the porphyrias. The technique is very quick and cost effective.

BLISTER FLUID

If you carefully remove the contents of a well selected blister, centrifuge some samples, or scrape the base or the roof of the blister, then you can create a useful slide with various histologic staining.

Special training is required, especially in reading slides. The technique is most useful in Zoster, varicella, herpes simplex, toxic epidermal necrolysis, scalded skin, some pyodermas, and urticaria pigmentosa.

No tests are in use using the chemistry of blister fluids.

ECTOPARASITES

Often you recover lice (three kinds), ticks or chiggers from the skin. Patients may bring in insects or arthropods that they suspect of harming them.

You can put lice in a small drop of oil on a slide under a cover slip for identification. Spiders or large insects are best put between two cotton balls in a small vial under 70% propanol to be sent for identification. Small bugs can be caught on scotch tape. Our experience is that people think they are being harmed by bites when they are not. Most specimens patients bring in are not biters. Your dermatologist is trained in medical entomology.

PATCH TESTING

▼ It is feasible to do testing for allergic contact dermatitis, both with crude products properly diluted or buffered, and with pure chemicals especially prepared for testing.

▼ Never test with materials not intended to be put on the skin, such as solvents or kitchen cleaners.

▼ Cosmetics can be tried on the skin of the inner arm to see that they are not harmful, prior to using them on the face. Proper dilutions may be needed to obtain reliable results.

▼ Also, photo-patch testing is available, requiring elaborate equipment and training.

▼ Some people have excessively irritable skin and must be tested with special materials.

▼ Tests will be falsely positive if the patient is tested too soon after the primary disease.

▼ Tests will be falsely negative if the patient is taking PO corticosteroids or using strong topical steroids. Patch tests can be suppressed by recent exposures to ultraviolet light.

TESTING FOR PHYSICAL URTICARIA

A series of standardized , readily repeatable, tests have been developed to examine allergy to cold, pressure, heat or light. These involve measurements and careful timing. The tests may be critical to optimal treatment. (Arrange these with your dermatologist).

SPECIAL TESTS FOR SKIN INFECTIONS

By gently crushing the tissue to produce an exudate, smears can be made that are better than biopsies. Leprosy and leishmaniasis are examples; most of the need is with rare disease.

Shallow shaves or cores of skin can be taken and quickly sectioned and stained to see the bacteria in necrotizing infections. This technique maximizes benefits until cultures are available. Early diagnosis may be life saving.

The dark-field technique to see spirochetes uses a special microscope with oblique lighting. To do this test is very labor intensive and expensive. Few patients with infectious syphilis today arrive at the clinic without having used some topical or systemic medicine that fouls the test. Scrupulous technique is required. Most centers no longer do the test, nor is it essential to proper care.

CULTURES FROM THE SKIN

Mostly, you are better advised to use a biopsy, alone or with the culture. Cultures from skin alone are notoriously unreliable. Almost all pyodermas are caused by mixed staphylococcus and streptococcus. Nothing is added by routine cultures of common pyodermas. Some clear justification is needed to culture bacteria from open skin.

> Cultures of herpes simplex should be done on atypical or controversial lesions, as early in the course of the eruption as possible.
> Cultures of tinea pedis or corporis are entirely for epidemiology. One should rely on the KOH examination for diagnosis.
> Cultures of tinea capitis are routinely useful in finding infections from house pets and because the KOH examination is difficult on the scalp.

BIOPSY OF SKIN

Try to use a standard 5mm punch biopsy technique for diagnosis. The procedure is a "clean-not sterile" procedure, and should be very simple and quick. Costs remain a concern but may be reduced. Use a modified procedure when needed. The key to skin biopsy is selection of the sample. Experience is valuable.

How to Punch

1. Choose carefully and prep lesion.
2. Inject 1% lidocaine, slowly and shallowly around the lesion for rapid effect and minimal injury to the specimen. Epinephrine will modify some vascular or granulomatous lesions.
3. Punch vertically to the plane of the skin, with a quick back and forth twisting motion, reaching in too fast. The plug should come free easily. Do not crush the plug in lifting it out. Snip the base, and put it in formalin solution.
4. As needed, close with 2 sutures of 4-0 or 5-0 suture.

Sampling Collaborate with you dermatologist. It is often useful to take 2 to 6 samples at the first examination of complex cases. Single specimens often bits are misleading. Try to pick a thick one, a thin one, old and new, center and margin. Or, take those of different primary lesions.

Doing the Histopathology

▼ Biopsy is only one laboratory test. The pathologist can not be expected to recognize the complexity of many cases. The clinician is responsible for the final diagnosis.

▼ All skin biopsies should be reviewed with your dermatologist.

▼ Errors are common place. Biopsies of the nose can falsely be read as basal cell carcinoma because of a concentration of hairs and follicles in odd patterns. Over reading, especially of melanocytic lesions, is a problem. Caution is advised. Don't accept histopathology as the SOLE support for an important diagnosis.

APPENDIX

CORTICOSTEROIDS (TOPICAL CREAM)

Listed by potency group. Group I is the most potent.

Group	Brand name	%	Generic name	Tube size (gm; unless noted)
I	Temovate cream	0.05	Clobetasol proprionate	15, 30, 45
	Temovate ointment	0.05		15, 30, 45
	Diprolene ointment	0.05		15, 45
	Diprolene AF cream	0.05	Betamethasone diproprionate	15, 45
	Psorcon ointment	0.05	Diflorasone diacelate	15, 30, 60
II	Alphatrex ointment	0.05	Betamethasone diproprionate	15, 45
	Cyclocon ointment	0.1	Amcinonide	15, 30, 60
	Diprosone ointment	0.05	Betamethasone diproprionate	15, 45
	Florone ointment	0.05	Diflorisone diacelate	15, 30, 60
	Halog (water solution) cream	0.1	Halcinonide	15, 30, 60, 240
	Halog ointment	0.1		15, 30, 60, 240
	Halog solution	0.1		20, 60 ml
	Halog-E cream	0.1		15, 30, 60
	Lidex (water solution) cream	0.05	Fluocinonide	15, 30, 60, 120
	Lidex gel	0.05		15, 30, 60, 120
	Lidex ointment	0.05		15, 30, 60, 120
	Lidex solution	0.05		20, 60 ml
	Lidex-E cream	0.05		15, 30, 60, 120
	Maxiflor ointment	0.05	Diflorasone diacetate	15, 30, 60
	Maxivate cream	0.05	Betamethasone dipropionate	15, 45
	Maxivate ointment	0.05		15, 45
	Topicort cream	0.25	Desoximetasone	15, 60, 120
	Topicort gel	0.05		15, 60

Group	Brand name	%	Generic name	Tube size (gm; unless noted)
III	Topicort ointment	0.25		15, 60
	Alphatrex cream	0.05	Betamethasone diproprionate	15, 45
	Alphatrex lotion	0.05		60 ml
	Aristocort cream	0.5	Triamcinolone acetonide	15, 240
	Aristocort ointment	0.5		15, 240
	Aristocort A cream	0.5		15, 240
	Benisone gel	0.025	Betamethasone benzoate	15, 60
	Betatrex ointment	0.1	Betamethasone valerate	15, 45
	Cyclocort lotion	0.1	Amcinonide	20, 60 ml
	Diprosone cream	0.05	Betamethasone diproprionate	15, 45
	Elcon ointment	0.1	Mometasone turoate	15, 45
	Florone cream	0.05	Diflorasone diacetate	15, 30, 60
	Florone E emollient	0.05		15, 30, 60
	Kenalog cream	0.5	Triamcinolone acetonide	20
	Kenalog ointment	0.5		20
	Maxiflor cream	0.05	Diflorasone diacetate	15, 30, 60
	Maxivate lotion	0.05	Betamethasone diproprionate	60 ml
	Trymex cream	0.5	Triamcinolone acetonide	15
	Uticort gel	0.025	Betamethasone benzoate	15, 60
	Uticort ointment	0.025		15, 60
	Valisone ointment	0.1	Betamethasone valerate	15, 45
IV	Aristocort ointment	0.1	Triamcinolone acetonide	15, 60, 240, 2400
	Benisone ointment	0.025	Betamethasone benzoate	15, 60
	Cordran ointment	0.05	Flurandrenolide	15, 30, 60, 225
	Cyclocort cream	0.1	Amcinonide	15, 30, 60

Group	Brand name	%	Generic name	Tube size (gm; unless noted)
	Elcon cream	0.1	Mometasene furoate	15, 45
	Elcon lotion	0.1		30, 60 ml
	Fluoride ointment	0.025	Fluocinolone acetonide	60
	Halog cream	0.025	Halcinonide	15, 60, 240
	Halog ointment	0.025		15, 60, 240
	Kenalog ointment	0.1	Triamcinolone acetonide	15, 60, 80, 240, 2520
	Synaler ointment	0.025	Fluocinolone acetonide	15, 30, 60, 120, 425
	Synalar-HP cream	0.2		12
	Topicort LP cream	0.05	Desoximetasone	15, 60
	Trymex ointment	0.1	Triamcinolone acetonide	15, 80
V	Aclovate cream	0.05	Alciometasone dipropionate	15, 45
	Aciovate ointment	0.05		15, 45
	Aristocort cream	0.1	Triamcinoione acetonide	15, 60, 240, 2520
	Benisone cream	0.025	Betamethasone benzoate	15, 60
	Beta-Val cream	0.1	Betamethasone valerate	15, 45
	Betatrex cream	0.1	Betamethasone valerate	15, 45
	Betatrex lotion	0.1		15, 60 ml
	Cloderm cream	0.1	Clocorcione pivalate	15, 45
	Cordran cream	0.05	Flurandrenolide	15, 30, 60, 225
	Cordran lotion	0.05		15, 60 ml
	Cordran ointment	0.025		30, 60, 225
	Deswen ointment	0.05	Desonide	15, 60
	Fluoride cream	0.025	Fluocinolone acetonide	15, 60
	Kenalog cream	0.1	Triamcinolone acetonide	15, 60, 80, 240, 2520

Group	Brand name	%	Generic name	Tube size (gm; unless noted)
	Kenalog lotion	0.1		15, 60 ml
	Kenalog ointment	0.025		15, 60, 80, 240
	Locoid cream	0.1	Hydrocortisone butyrate	15, 45, 60
	Locoid ointment	0.1		15, 45, 2520
	Synalar cream	0.025	Fluocinolone acetonide	15, 30, 60, 425
	Synemol cream	0.025	Fluocinolone acetonide	15, 30, 60
	Tridesilon ointment	0.05	Desonide	15, 60
	Trymex cream	0.1	Triamcinolone acetonide	15, 80, 480
	Trymex ointment	0.025		15, 80
	Uticort cream	0.025	Betamethasone benzoate	15, 60
	Uticort lotion	0.025		15, 60 ml
	Valisone cream	0.1	Betamethasone valerate	15, 45, 110, 430
	Valisone lotion	0.1		20, 60 ml
	Westcort cream	0.2	Hydrocortisone	15, 45, 60, 120
	Westcort ointment	0.2		15, 45, 60
VI	Aristocort cream	0.025	Triamcinolone acetonide	15, 60, 240, 2520
	Deswen cream	0.05	Desonide	15, 60
	Fluonid cream	0.01	Fluocinotone acetonide	15, 60
	Fluonid solution	0.01		20, 60 ml
	Kenalog cream	0.025	Triamcinolone acetonide	15, 60, 80, 240, 2520
	Kenalog lotion	0.025		60 ml
	Locorten cream	0.03	Flumethasone pivolate	15, 60
	Synalar cream	0.01	Flucoinolone acetonide	15, 45, 60, 425
	Synalar solution	0.01		20, 60 ml
	Tridesilon cream	0.05	Desonide	15, 60

continued

Group	Brand name	%	Generic name	Tube size (gm; unless noted)
	Trymex cream	0.025	Triamcinolone acetonide	15, 80, 480
	Valisone cream	0.01	Betamethasone valerate	15, 60
VII	Celestone cream	0.2	Betamethasone valerate	15
	Decaderm gel	0.1	Dexamethasone	15, 30
	Hytone cream	1.0	Hydrocortisone	1, 4 oz
		2.5		1, 2 oz
	Hytone lotion	1.0		4 oz
		2.5		2 oz
	Hytone ointment	1.0		1, 4 oz
		2.5		1 oz
	Lacticare lotion	1.0	Hydrocortisone	4 oz
		2.5		2 oz
	Medrol cream	0.25	Methylprednisolone	7.5, 30, 45
	Oxylone cream	0.025	Fluoromethalone	15, 60, 120
	Synacort cream	1.0	Hydrocortisone	15, 30, 60
		2.5		30

INDEX

Page numbers in italics denote figures; those followed by a t denote tables.

5-Fluorouracil, for actinic dermatitis, 313
6-Methylcoumcum, photoallergy
 from, 269t

ABCD criteria, for melanoma, 156–157
ABCDT criteria, for nevi, 77–78, 80, 81
Abnormalities. *See* Birth defects
Acantholysis, from pemphigus, 219, 221
Accinthocytes, in herpes simplex, 70
Accutane. *See* Isotretinoin
ACE inhibitors, urticaria and
 angioedema from, 105
Acetaminophen
 for herpes zoster (shingles), 215
 for infectious mononucleosis, 204
 for viral exanthems, 205
Acetocholine, in cholinergic
 urticaria, 104
Acetowhitening, for genital warts, 114
Acetylsalicylic acid, for sunburn, 264
Aclovate. *See* Alclometasone
 dipropionate
Acne
 acute conglobate, 28
 from anabolic steroids, 320
 antibiotics for, 24
 irritant, 39
 mechanica, 315, 318
 nodulocystic, 38
 rosacea. *See* Rosacea
 vs. perifolliculitis capitis, 322
 vulgaris, 35–42, 36, *41*
  case study, 41
  diagnosis of, 36–37
  etiology and symptoms, 35, 39
  grades of, 36–39
  patient education for, 42
  prognosis for, 39
  treatment of, 36–37
Acneiform diseases, 16
Acquired immunodeficiency syndrome.
 See AIDS
Acrodermatitis chronica atrophicus,
 from lyme borreliosis, 285t, 287

Acrodermatitis enteropathica, from zinc
 deficiency, 327
Actinic keratosis. *See* Keratosis, actinic
Actinic poikiloderma. *See* Poikiloderma,
 actinic
Acyclovir
 for chicken pox, 212
 for genital herpes simplex, 26
 for herpes genitalis, 73
 for herpes simplex, 70, 71
 for herpes zoster, 26
 for herpes zoster (shingles), 208
 for labial herpes simplex, 26
 for varicella zoster, 26, 27
Addison's disease, vitiligo and, 174
Adolescents. *See* Children and
 adolescents
Adrenal cortex hormones.
 See Corticosteroids
African-Americans, skin diseases and,
 320–323
Age and aging
 actinic dermatitis and, 312–313
 alopecia and, 312
 basal cell carcinoma and, 253
 pemphigoid and, 225
 pemphigus and, 222
 photosensitivity and, 271
 pressure sores and, 311
 pruritus with, 182–183
 purpura with, 240
 seborrheic dermatitis and, 311
 seborrheic keratosis and, 313
 skin diseases and, 308–313
 sunburn and, 262
 wound healing and, 311
Agency for Health Care Policy and
 Research, 309
AIDS. *See also* HIV
 seborrheic dermatitis with, 99
 squamous cell carcinoma with, 258t
Airway maintenance, for insect bites
 and stings, 147, 150
Albinism
 with basal cell carcinoma, 249

Mast cell degranulation
in pemphigoid, 222
urticaria and angioedema from, 104, 105
Mastocytosis multiple myelinoma,
pruritus from, 184t
Maternal-fetal exchange, herpes simplex
from, 70
Maxiflor. *See* Diflorasone diacetate
Maxivate. *See* Betamethasone
dipropionate
Measles, 16, 197–198
vs. rubella, 198
Medical entomology, 330
Medical history taking, 12, 29
Medication. *See also* Antibiotics;
Antifungals; Antihistamines;
Antivirals; Corticosteroids; Names
of individual drugs; Nonsteroidal
anti-inflammatory drugs; Steroids
topical, 29–30, 334t–338t
Medrol. *See* Methylprednisolone
Medroxyprogesterone acetate, acne
vulgaris from, 35, 40
Melanin
in sunburn, 262
Wood's light for, 329
Melanocyte simulating hormone, during
pregnancy, 76
Melanocytes
with basal cell carcinoma, 249
in sunburn, 263, 265
Melanoma, 154–162, *160*
biopsy for, 79
in black patients, 322
from blistering sunburn, 265
case study, 160–161
color of, 13
diagnosis of, 15, 154–158
etiology and symptoms, 154–157
mortality from, 154
nail bed, 168
from nevi, 76–77
patient education for, 162
prognosis for, 156, 159
screening for, 155–158
vs. dermatofibromas, 134
vs. photoaging, 267
vs. pigmented basal cell carcinoma, 253
vs. seborrheic keratosis, 141
vs. talon noir, 317
Melasma. *See* Chloasma
Meningitis, from lyme borreliosis,
285t, 287
Meningococcemia, vs. exanthems, 201

Menthol,
for allergic contact dermatitis, 52
Metastasis. *See* Cancer, metastasis
Methotrexate, 24
alopecia from, 126
hair loss from, 245
nail dystrophies from, 245
for pemphigus, 221
for psoriasis of the nails, 166, 169
for pustular psoriasis, 85
Methylprednisolone, 338t
Metronidazole, for rosacea,
191, 192, 193
Micrographic surgery. *See* Mohs surgery
Miliaria, 16
in neonates, 300–301
vs. exanthems, 202
Mineral oil, application of, 30
Minocycline
for acne, 24
for acne vulgaris, 37, 39
hyperpigmentation from, 245
Minoxidil, for pattern baldness, 125, 128
Mohs surgery
for basal cell carcinoma, 251, 252
for squamous cell carcinoma, 251, 257
Moisturizers. *See* Lubricants
Moles. *See* Nevi
Molluscum contagiosum,
15, 138–139, 142
Mometasone furoate, 31, 335t
Mongolian spots, in neonates, 302–303
Morphea, necrobiosis lipoidicum
diabeticum and, 298
Morphine, pruritus from, 184t
Mouth, examination of, 21
MSH. *See* Melanocyte simulating
hormone
Mucous membranes
blisters from pemphigus, 220
examination of, 19–20, 21
iron deficiency and, 326
malnutrition and, 323–324
in pemphigoid, 223
squamous cell carcinoma of,
255–256, 258
Myocarditis, from Rocky Mountain
spotted fever, 290
Myocelitis, with measles, 198
Myopericarditis, from lyme borreliosis,
285t, 287

Nails
care of in diabetes, 300